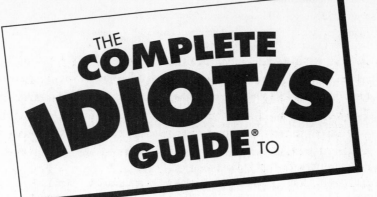

THE COMPLETE IDIOT'S GUIDE® TO

Getting a Tattoo

D0112061

by John Reardon

ALPHA

A member of Penguin Group (USA) Inc.

ALPHA BOOKS

391.65
R234c

Published by the Penguin Group

Penguin Group (USA) Inc., 375 Hudson Street, New York, New York 10014, USA

Penguin Group (Canada), 90 Eglinton Avenue East, Suite 700, Toronto, Ontario M4P 2Y3, Canada (a division of Pearson Penguin Canada Inc.)

Penguin Books Ltd., 80 Strand, London WC2R 0RL, England

Penguin Ireland, 25 St. Stephen's Green, Dublin 2, Ireland (a division of Penguin Books Ltd.)

Penguin Group (Australia), 250 Camberwell Road, Camberwell, Victoria 3124, Australia (a division of Pearson Australia Group Pty. Ltd.)

Penguin Books India Pvt. Ltd., 11 Community Centre, Panchsheel Park, New Delhi—110 017, India

Penguin Group (NZ), 67 Apollo Drive, Rosedale, North Shore, Auckland 1311, New Zealand (a division of Pearson New Zealand Ltd.)

Penguin Books (South Africa) (Pty.) Ltd., 24 Sturdee Avenue, Rosebank, Johannesburg 2196, South Africa

Penguin Books Ltd., Registered Offices: 80 Strand, London WC2R 0RL, England

International Standard Book Number: 978-1-59257-725-5
Library of Congress Catalog Card Number: 2007906890

10   09   08   8   7   6   5   4   3   2   1

Interpretation of the printing code: The rightmost number of the first series of numbers is the year of the book's printing; the rightmost number of the second series of numbers is the number of the book's printing. For example, a printing code of 08-1 shows that the first printing occurred in 2008.

Printed in the United States of America

Note: This publication contains the opinions and ideas of its author. It is intended to provide helpful and informative material on the subject matter covered. It is sold with the understanding that the author and publisher are not engaged in rendering professional services in the book. If the reader requires personal assistance or advice, a competent professional should be consulted.

The author and publisher specifically disclaim any responsibility for any liability, loss, or risk, personal or otherwise, which is incurred as a consequence, directly or indirectly, of the use and application of any of the contents of this book.

Most Alpha books are available at special quantity discounts for bulk purchases for sales promotions, premiums, fund-raising, or educational use. Special books, or book excerpts, can also be created to fit specific needs.

For details, write: Special Markets, Alpha Books, 375 Hudson Street, New York, NY 10014.

Publisher: *Marie Butler-Knight*
Editorial Director: *Mike Sanders*
Managing Editor: *Billy Fields*
Senior Acquisitions Editor: *Paul Dinas*
Development Editor: *Nancy D. Lewis*
Senior Production Editor: *Janette Lynn*
Copy Editor: *Jan Zoya*

Cartoonist: *Shannon Wheeler*
Cover Designer: *Bill Thomas*
Book Designer: *Trina Wurst*
Indexer: *Heather McNeill*
Layout: *Brian Massey*
Proofreader: *Aaron Black*

This book is dedicated to the loving memory of John Paras. He was a great tattooist and a best friend. He was there when you needed help.

Contents at a Glance

Contents

Appendixes

Foreword

Tattoos hurt. There's no two ways about it.

I was 17 years old when I walked into my first tattoo shop. My palms were sweaty, my knees trembling, and I had knots in my stomach. I was set on getting the words "DRUG FREE" tattooed on my back. Once I was lying down and the letters were drawn on, I heard the buzz of the machine. I took a deep breath and felt the sting of the needle as the first line was made. For a moment, I thought to myself, "I might not be able to handle this." I thought I might be one of those people you hear about, walking around with half an outline of a tattoo, forever marked with a badge of shame, showing the world that I wasn't tough enough to sit through a tattoo. Then I realized that the pain was in fact bearable. It wasn't that bad at all. I began to relax and get more comfortable. As I lay there, my tattoo slowly came together. It began to scratch an itch I never knew I had. By the time the artist finished, I wanted more. I was hooked.

Now, 12 years later, I've been tattooing for the past 7 years. I owe my career in large part to John Reardon. John started to teach me to tattoo in the fall of 1998. We were both attending Pratt Institute of Art in Brooklyn, and John was busy working at a tattoo shop on St. Mark's Place in Manhattan. There wasn't a lot of time for him to show me the proverbial ropes. Needless to say, by the time I did my first tattoo out of my dorm room, I was more nervous than the client about to get stuck with needles. John watched over my shoulder as I shakily lined a fraternity symbol on an acquaintance of mine. He was eager to get tattooed, and obviously not very particular about how the tattoo looked. Learning how to tattoo out of my dorm room was slow-going, so John managed to pull some strings and get me an apprenticeship at the tattoo shop where he was working. I spent the next year learning the basics of tattooing and sterilization under the supervision of John, along with Tanya "Pinky" Goldberg, Eddy Molina, and Miki Fogged. By early 2000, I got my first job tattooing professionally.

Since then, tattooing has changed so much. It's remarkable to me. I can only imagine how it must be to some of the tattooists who have seen it evolve. What was once an art form for sailors, bikers, outlaws, and misfits in general, is now something accepted by all walks of life. Tattoos are everywhere nowadays. Wildly accepted in pop-culture, there are numerous television shows about tattooing. Kmart even sells teen clothing covered in tattoo imagery. Tattooing has gone from something that was looked down upon by society to an art form that nearly everyone wants to collect a small piece of. I've even been yelled at by a mother for *not* tattooing her 15-year-old daughter!

Poor parenting aside, that's why this book is such a good idea. The problem is that it's hard for the tattoo client to know what to look for. The point of this book is to give you some inside knowledge as to who is worth getting tattooed by. There are a lot of great tattoo artists out there, but there are a lot more horrible ones. This book will also give you an idea of what kind of imagery might be better suited for a tattoo. I spend a good amount of my day explaining to people that a tattoo needs an outline and black shading to hold up over the years. Trust me, I wish there had been *The Complete Idiot's Guide to Getting a Tattoo* when I first started getting tattooed. It would have changed some of the decisions I made, and I'd be happier with my earlier tattoos.

On television, t-shirts, billboards, and nearly every body, tattooing is everywhere today. Clients are coming into tattoo shops better prepared with images they've researched in magazines, books, and on the Internet. They're more trusting of the artist they've chosen because they've taken the time to look into who they want to be tattooed by. Overall, the tattooing world is in a good place and seems to be getting better. New generations of tattooists are coming up and creating some really impressive tattoos.

So the next time you're ready to get a tattoo, think back to the lessons you've learned in this book, and choose wisely. Good luck.

—Eli S. Quinters

Eli graduated from Pratt Institute of Art in 2001, with a BFA in Illustration. Since February of 2007, Eli has tattooed out of a private studio in Williamsburg, Brooklyn. You can see his work at www.tattoosfortheunloved.com.

Introduction

If you have picked up this book, you are either going to get your first tattoo or getting prepared for another one. Here is your opportunity to learn about tattooing and how to get a good tattoo so you don't end up with an embarrassing mess. Tattooing is becoming more and more popular with TV shows such as *Miami Ink*. Many celebrities and professional athletes can be seen sporting fresh tattoos on TV all the time. You most likely have at least one friend or acquaintance who has a tattoo. Now it's your turn.

This book will guide you through the process of getting a tattoo. Many people find that a tattoo shop can be an intimidating place. We will go over the various aspects of tattoo shops so you will feel more comfortable when you go in for your tattoo. You will see what to look for when choosing a good tattooist to ensure that you are happy with your tattoo.

What You'll Learn in This Book

In order to make your understanding of the world of tattooing come easily, we have divided the book into three parts.

In **Part 1, "What Is a Tattoo?"** we go over the history of tattoos through the various origins of the different styles. We cover how tattoos are viewed in society and how that is changing. We then go over the most popular styles of tattoo design that have emerged over the years. We then go into the scientific aspects of how tattoos stay in the skin. We continue with what is used to make the tattoo and the different ways tattooing can be done. We then follow up with the formalities of tattooing and some of the reasons why a person may not be able to get a tattoo.

In **Part 2, "Beginning the Tattoo Process,"** we start to look at what aspects a tattoo design needs in order for the design to be tattooed. We will check out how to choose the tattooist who is right for you. Not all tattooists know what they are doing. We will see how to determine the quality of a tattooist's work so you will have a clean tattoo.

In **Part 3, "Get in the Chair,"** you will see how to prepare yourself so that you will be comfortable while you are getting tattooed. We will cover the ins and outs of the tattoo shop, from its set-up to the people you will meet there. We will get down to the actual process of getting a tattoo so you can see what you will experience. Then we will go over what you need to do after the tattoo is complete and what to do if you need a tattoo removed or covered.

Extras

I've developed a few helpers you'll find in little boxes throughout this book:

def•i•ni•tion

Terms you will hear in a tattoo shop—they will help you to understand the tattoo process.

Inkformation

Interesting historical or trivia facts about tattoos and how to make the most of your tattoo experience.

Tat-tale

Interesting anecdotes about tattoos.

Tattoo Taboo

Warnings about tattoos and the tattoo experience.

Flash Tip

Hints on getting more out of the tattoo experience.

Acknowledgments

I would not have had the opportunity to write this book if it was not for my sister, Wendy Reardon, who wrote *The Complete Idiot's Guide to Exotic and Pole Dancing*. She hooked me up with this gig by introducing me to her—and now my—editor Paul Dinas. I would like to thank Mr. Dinas for all his patience, guidance, and most important, kicking my derrière to make sure this project was completed practically on time.

I would like to thank my beautiful wife, Amina Reardon, for her support and understanding. Thanks to my parents, John and Joan Reardon, for popping me out and giving me drive to do more with my life. Thanks to Beth Reardon Hughes and her husband Neal Hughes for keeping track of my progress and encouraging me to finish. Thanks to Eli Quinters for helping me out by allowing me to use his tattoo photos and flash, and for being a good influence and a great friend.

Thanks to Bryce Ward (www.bryceward.com) who is responsible for the majority of the photographs in this book.

Thank you everyone at Saved Tattoo for the support and understanding of me not being around or just running around frantic, Scott Campbell, Dan Trocchio, Othello Gervacio, Beau Valasco, Joseph Ari Aloi (JK5), Michelle Tarantelli (thanks for the help with the skin illustrations, you rule), Brody, James O'Brien, and the huggable Myles Karr. I would also like to thank my clientele for being patient with me when I was not really able to tattoo them while I was writing this book. It's on now.

Thanks to Shinji, Steve Bolts, Burt Krak, Chad Koeplinger, D'Joe, Steve Byrne, Amina Reardon, Dan Trocchio, Michelle Tarentelli, Scott Campbell, Joseph Ari Aloi (JK5), Myles Karr, Thomas Hooper, Mathew Amey (Skull Project), Brian (Awake One), Tyler Densley, Chris O'Donnell, Mike Rubendall, and Henning Jorgensen for the use of their tattoo photos. Thanks to Shag (Mike Kruse) at Revenant Publishing, for organizing a bunch of flash sheets. Thanks to everyone who sent in flash. I hope this book gives you all more clients who want to get fun tattoos in your individual preferred styles.

Trademarks

Part 1

What Is a Tattoo?

Getting a tattoo can be a wonderful experience or a nerve-racking experience. The best way to make your first tattoo a good experience is to understand what is going on during the procedure.

In this part, we will go over the history of tattooing and its social significance. You will learn how tattoos work and what is being used to create them.

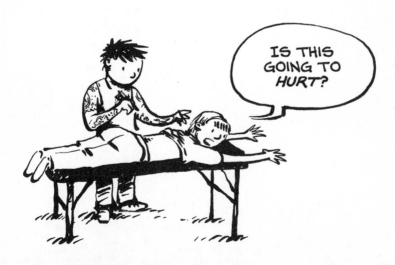

The Beginning of Tattoos

In This Chapter

- ◆ Early origins of tattooing
- ◆ How tribal tattoos influenced the Western world
- ◆ The development of modern tattooing
- ◆ What is happening today with tattooing

Tattooing is probably one of the few professions that has been around longer than prostitution. Tattooing has had the same amount of persecution, if not more. Evidence of tattoo implements has been found in Europe, and dates back between 10,000 and 30,000 B.C.E. If your parents or grandparents want to give you grief for getting a tattoo, you can remind them that further back in the family tree, by a few thousand years, your ancestors were most likely getting tattooed by the campfire. That probably won't dissuade them, but at least you tried.

This chapter talks about the origins of tattooing. You will see how the designs of today are based on what tribes have done in the past. You will learn how tattooing developed into what it is today so that when you are ready for your tattoo, it will mean something more than just a permanent sticker would.

The South Pacific; Polynesia

The Polynesian Islands are located in the South Pacific. They stretch from Hawaii to Easter Island to New Zealand. The tattooing in Polynesia is considered the most beautiful and mastered of ancient tattooing. The people of the Polynesian Islands are known for having large tattoos, often covering their faces. Unfortunately, due to western globalization in the nineteenth century, tattooing was banned on many islands. This led to the loss of many tattooing traditions and designs.

The Marquesian Islands lie 1,200 miles west of Peru. The ancient Marquesians developed an ornate style of tattooing that can cover most of the body. The designs are geometric patterns and images, which fit well to the body.

Borneo

Borneo is the third-largest island in the world after Greenland and New Guinea. It is perhaps because of its size that Borneo has been left mostly untouched by the Western world. The inland tribes who have little or no contact with the outside world have had their traditional way of life preserved. Many of their tattoo designs are hundreds of years old and are still tattooed today.

Maori

The Maori are the native people of New Zealand. The Maori are famous for the Moko, a facial tattoo. This beautiful tattoo is a representation of its wearer. The Moko portrays the individual's social status and is, in a sense, the wearer's signature. These tattoos are "carved" into the face of the wearer, leaving a ridge-like scar. A good example of the Moko can be seen in the film *Once Were Warriors*, directed by Lee Tamahori.

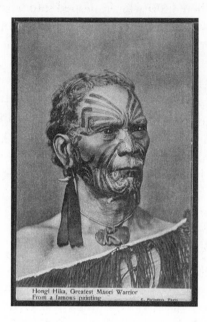

Maori tattoo.

(Photo courtesy of Tattoo Archive)

Hawaii

The traditional tattooing in Hawaii is called "Kakau." Not only were tattoos for decorating the body, but they were also used for physical and spiritual protection. The designs also portrayed an individual's social status.

Samoa

Tatau is the Samoan word for tattoo. The word tatau is actually the origin of the western word tattoo. The Samoan tattoo is very important in portraying social class. It is a very elaborate affair when the son of a chief is tattooed. The Samoan tattoo usually covers the lower torso down to the knee, like a pair of shorts. The process of getting this tattoo would usually begin at the start of puberty, marking the beginning of adulthood.

Africa

Most of African-body modification relies on *scarification*. Scarification is purposefully creating a scar in the skin for decoration. Ancient Egypt, however, had its own form of tattooing. Egyptologists have found written records dealing with tattoos and works of art seemingly decorated with tattoos. A female body from the XI Dynasty was found in 1891 bearing many lines and dashes, which formed abstract geometric patterns. These tattoos were probably used for certain religious rituals.

def•i•ni•tion

Scarification is the act of scarring the skin to make a pattern or design.

North and South America

Tattooing was an important cultural part of the tribes of the Americas. As with the Polynesian tribes, tattooing among American tribes came to represent social status as well as marks of victory over an enemy. Tattooing was also used in the ritual of beginning adulthood. Unfortunately, most of the indigenous societies were destroyed and their traditions banned and lost.

Some examples of traditional tattooing found in North America are:

◆ The Iroquois were tattooed to show social status. The larger and more ornate the tattoo, the higher the status an individual had.

◆ The Haida of the northwest were tattooed with designs that represented family heritage. These designs were of animals, similar to the popular totem-pole designs.

◆ The women of the Inuit people in the northwest had their chins tattooed to represent their marital status.

Much of the evidence of tattooing in South America is found in the writings of the conquistadors, the Spanish explorers, between the fifteenth and seventeenth centuries. The Spanish had never seen tattooing before and, being devout Catholics, considered it the work of the devil. The Spanish thought it was bad enough that the natives worshipped "demonic" statues, but were disgusted when they saw the natives had managed to print these images on their bodies.

In Mayan society, the wealthy were elaborately tattooed to show their social status. A good example of this can be seen in Mel Gibson's *Apocolypto*. Unfortunately, the conquistadors destroyed much of the indigenous culture of South and Central America.

Inkformation

A well-preserved 5,000-year-old body was found frozen in the Tyrolean Alps, between Italy and Austria. The well-preserved skin of the mummified specimen showcased the body's 57 tattoos. The body had many parallel lines tattooed on the ankles, and six straight lines, each 15 centimeters long, above the kidneys. The body also had a cross tattooed on the inside of the left knee. The placement of the tattoos implies they were placed on the specific parts of the body for therapeutic reasons. The tattoos were possibly an early treatment of arthritis. If you would like to see this mummy, it is on display at the South Tyrol Museum in Bolzano, Italy.

Japan

Japanese tattooing has had an enormous influence on modern tattooing. Sailors would come back from Japan with intricate dragons and other Japanese designs. Western tattooists copied these designs or had the designs tattooed on them when they were in the Navy. It can be said that the old western style of tattooing came together with Japanese tattooing to create the modern tattoo design.

Many western tattooists specialize in Japanese-style tattooing. Some western tattooists have even learned the traditional "hand poke" technique of Japanese tattooing.

The Ainu

The Ainu are a tribal group of people who live mainly on the island of Hokkaido, the second-largest island located in northern Japan. The Ainu have inhabited Japan for over ten thousand years and many have integrated into modern Japanese society. The Ainu woman would have their arms, mouths, and sometimes their foreheads tattooed. This would usually occur at the start of puberty.

Criminal Markings

In the seventh century, the rulers of Japan came to adopt their attitude toward tattooing from the Chinese. Tattooing was considered barbaric and only used as a form of punishment.

Inkformation

This chapter covers only a very brief history of tattooing. If you would like to learn more, check out *The Tattoo History Source Book* by Steve Gilbert (PowerHouse Books, 2001).

In 720 C.E., an emperor sentenced a man to be tattooed as a worse form of punishment than to be put to death. The Japanese had perfected a system of tattoo markings for criminals to show their crime. This put the criminals in the lowest social class and ostracized the criminal from his or her friends and family.

By the end of the seventeenth century, decorative tattooing began to become popular again. Penal tattoos were then covered up with other designs. This is perhaps the start of tattoos in Japan being fully connected with organized crime. At the same time that tattooing was becoming popular, tattooing as a punishment started to be replaced with other forms of punishment.

Japanese Prints as Influence

By the eighteenth century, tattooing started to draw influence from wood-block prints of images called "ukiyoe," or "pictures of the floating world." One of the most famous and influential ukiyoe artists was Kuniyoshi (1798–1861).

Kuniyoshi illustrated one of the most popular stories of the time, the *Suikoden*. The Suikoden originated in China and is a story of 108 outlaws who defied the corrupt rulers of China. Many of them were tattooed. These characters were very popular for over a century, and the illustrations of the tattooed warriors are still a major influence on tattooing today.

Some of the original clients of Japanese tattooists were firefighters. They would bare their tattoos as a sign of courage while battling fires. The yakuza, or Japanese mafia, kept the tradition of tattooing as well. To this day, many *bodysuits* in Japan are on yakuza.

def•i•ni•tion

A **bodysuit** refers to having your body covered with tattoos.

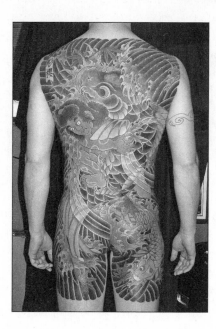

Tattoo by Shinji (Horizakura), New York Adorned, Brooklyn, NY, www.nyadorned.com.

The Beginning of Modern Electric Tattooing

The sailors who came into contact with the different tattoo cultures began to collect tattoos themselves. They started to tattoo each other, by hand, and brought the craft back home. Different designs for tattoos were being created and kept in the studios for reuse. These designs came to be known as *flash*. England was a popular spot for tattooing because many naval officers would get tattooed, as well as British royalty. Hori Chyo tattooed the Duke of York in Yokohama in 1882; the Duke of York later became King George V.

def•i•ni•tion

Tattoo designs that are created for multiple uses are known as **flash**. Typically they are displayed in the tattoo shop in flash racks, on the wall, or in books.

The popularity of tattooing in England spread and soon there were tattoo shops in every port. Tattooing was imported to U.S. ports where it flourished in New York. It was in New York where the advent of electricity modernized the tattoo process.

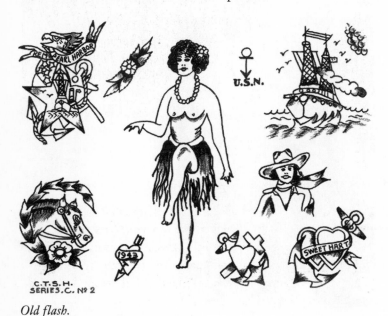

Old flash.

(Photo courtesy of Tattoo Archive)

The First Machine

In 1891, a New Yorker named Samuel O'Reilly patented the first electric tattoo machine. O'Reilly had been tattooing by hand on the infamous Bowery (Third Avenue) in lower Manhattan. He took an electric rotary engraving device created by Thomas Edison and modified it so it could be used for tattooing. O'Reilly soon offered the device for sale, along with designs, colors, and other tattoo supplies. This created a boom of new tattooists.

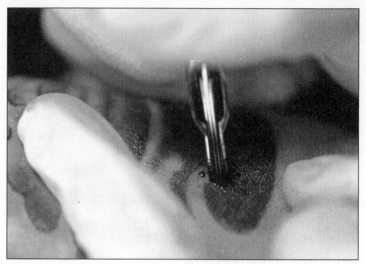

Tattoo up close.

The Circus

In the nineteenth century, circuses started using heavily tattooed people as part of the "Freak Show." Some of the sailors would come back from Polynesia, covered in tattoos. The mainstream Western world had never seen that before and would pay to see the tattooed "freaks." Some heavily tattooed people even had audiences with the various royal families of Europe.

In 1842, P. T. Barnum employed James F. O'Connell as the first tattooed man ever on exhibit in the United States. Many circuses also employed tattooists to tattoo the circus goers. Places like Coney Island became hotspots for tattooing.

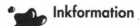 **Inkformation**

Freak Show exhibits included strange and unusual things such as bearded ladies, two-headed cows, heavily tattooed people, fire eaters, and sword swallowers.

The Sailor Tattoo

In the early twentieth century, tattooing primarily flourished in the ports of major cities such as New York and Copenhagen. Sailors would spend their money on booze and tattoos. The designs usually consisted of pin-up girls, sailing ships, roses, anchors, and hearts, to name a few. Tattooists would see tattoos from other tattooists in different countries. It wasn't long before tattooists began to contact each other.

Sailor Jerry Collins was a tattooist working in Honolulu and was contacted by the Japanese tattooist Kazuo Oguri in 1970. The two traded information, such as where to get good colors as well as design concepts. Sailor Jerry was also in contact with two younger tattooists, Mike Malone and Ed Hardy. Soon Kazuo Oguri was introduced to Malone and Hardy, and a bridge between Japanese tattooing and western tattooing was built.

The Tattoo Convention

Tattooists have traditionally been very secretive, but by the mid '70s, tattooists started to get together. Tattooists started to organize tattoo conventions. The conventions became meeting grounds for tattooists to share ideas, show their work, and drink together. Bonds were formed and tattooists began to visit each other, working in each other's shops. Conventions also allowed for tattoo enthusiasts to get tattooed by someone who lived in another state or country. Today there are tattoo conventions all the time, all over the world.

> **Tat-tale**
>
> One of the first international tattoo conventions was held in Amsterdam. It consisted of seven tattooists, one of them being Tato Svend of Copenhagen, Denmark, all sitting around a small dark bar and tattooing one guy.

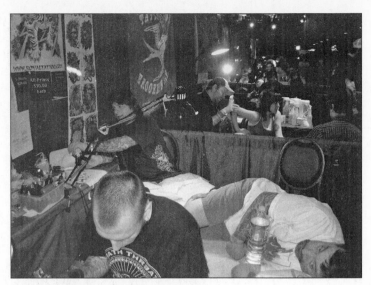

New York City Tattoo convention.

Famous Patrons

The lore of tattooing knows no bound. Throughout history, many western monarchs have been tattooed. Today, pop stars and professional athletes are covered in tattoos and often show them off to the cameras for all to see. Let's look at a few historical, famous patrons who paved the way for social acceptance of the art.

- ◆ King Frederick IX of Denmark (1899–1972). King Frederick was the King of Denmark from 1947 to 1972. As a sailor, King Frederick was heavily tattooed and thus reinforced the tradition of sailors having tattoos and Nyhavn, Copenhagen as a hot spot for getting them.

- ◆ The Great Omi (1892–1969). The great Omi was a British army officer before becoming one of the world's most famous "Barbaric Beauties."

- ◆ King George V (1865–1936). In 1882, when King George was still a duke, he was tattooed by Hori Chyo.

The Great Omi.

(Photo courtesy of Tattoo Archive)

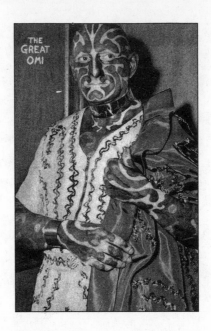

Tattoo Commercialism

Tattooing has become so popular and socially accepted that it has become highly marketable. *Miami Ink*, a reality TV show about a tattoo shop on South Beach, has broadened the acceptance of tattooing. Many corporations such as Camel cigarettes are using tattoo designs in their advertisement campaigns to reach customers. Ed Hardy, one of the pioneers of tattooing, even has his own energy drink and clothing line. Christian Audigier, who also made Von Dutch a household name, runs Ed Hardy Vintage Tattoo Wear. Ed Hardy Vintage Tattoo Wear is geared toward high-end fashion and has numerous pop stars such as Lil Jon featured in its advertisements.

Inkformation

If you don't want to wear a tattoo on your skin, you can always just buy a t-shirt. Many tattooists have their designs printed on t-shirts or sweatshirts and sell them online. Sailor Jerry Limited makes products, from t-shirts and jackets to aprons and ashtrays, branded with the old master's designs.

Prints and Paintings

To be a great tattooist, you have to be a great artist. Many tattooists are involved in other mediums such as oil or ink painting. This gives tattooists another way to express themselves and an opportunity to work on a canvas that doesn't move. If you can't get a tattoo, you can always buy it as a painting or print.

At events such as The New York City Upstarts Show (held every year in May during the NYC Tattoo Convention) or in stores like Tattoo Elite International, fans buy prints from amazing tattooists such as Mike Rubendall and Henning Jorgensen. Prints are great because they won't break your bank account to purchase, but you can still have a beautiful piece of artwork to hang on your wall.

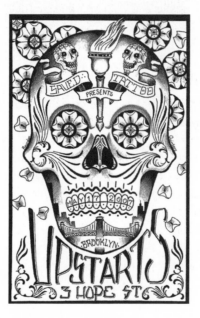

Poster for the 2007 annual New York City Upstarts Show.

The Least You Need to Know

- Tattooing has been a part of human culture for over 10,000 years.

- In tribal cultures, tattooing was used to show the social status of an individual.

- The beginning of western tattooing came from the sailors who explored the South Pacific.

- Sailor Jerry Collins and Ed Hardy played an important role in the modernization of tattooing by building international correspondences.

- Tattooing is becoming more of a fine art with the development of custom tattoos and the buying and selling of tattoo-influenced art.

Chapter 2

Tattoos and Society

In This Chapter

◆ The changing attitude toward tattoos

◆ What it means to have large tattoos

◆ When tattooing goes overboard

◆ What the military thinks about tattoos

As we have seen in the previous chapter, tattoos have long been a meaningful part of society. Tattoos have been embraced by cultures and used to define an individual's status, whether it be a chief's son or a Japanese lawbreaker. Even if you just want a cute little butterfly on your shoulder, that tattoo will mean something to someone.

In this chapter, we will explore the social aspects of tattooing. We will discuss the attitudes different cultures have had toward tattooing and how those have affected today's growing acceptance of tattoos.

Old Attitudes

Much of the western religious philosophies deem it sacrilegious to alter the human body. In Leviticus 19:28, the King James version, there is a mention to making body marks, "Ye shall not make any cuttings in your flesh for the dead, nor print any marks upon you …." One must agree that to ban something in a culture, the culture must be doing it in the first place. Thus, tattooing was a part of the culture at that time.

In the race to spread monotheism, Jewish and Christian leaders connected tattooing with heathen polytheists. Tattooing in Europe and the Middle East at that time was done mainly for religious and superstitious reasons. Tattooing was relatively widespread among tribal people. In order to keep people from believing in anything that wasn't monotheistic in nature, any form of tattooing that didn't show a devotion to God was looked at as sacrilegious.

Over time, as the control of Christianity became stronger, religious leaders saw all tattooing as the work of heathens. It was the Roman emperor, Constantine, who banned tattooing because he thought it was "un-Christian." This attitude made tattooing very unpopular in the Western world. Tattoos were associated with those who were "unholy" and not likely to receive "God's blessing."

Later it was the crusaders and then the pilgrims who wanted to spread Christianity through exploration. When they would reach Jerusalem, the Christian Crusaders would get a tattoo as a sign of devotion and to mark this memorable journey, not unlike the exploring sailors who eventually ventured to the Polynesian Islands and got tattooed by the local inhabitants.

As Christian nations started to conquer and pillage foreign soil, they needed to break the hearts and minds of the peoples they conquered to make them easier to control. What worked at home would certainly work in these new lands. The Christian religion and all of its rules and regulations were forced upon the conquered peoples. Tattooing in most of the colonized islands was banned.

The heathens, who seemed to have done just fine over the previous thousands of years, were "saved" and brought to Christianity. This was just a tool to strip the people of their identity, breaking their spirit and their ability to stand up for themselves. It worked just as well as England's divide-and-conquer routine (the act of getting two local factions to war with each other in order to make both factions weak and easier to conquer), in breaking the natives' spirits. Not to mention that smallpox and other devastating diseases brought by the westerners killed off many. In 1887, the French took a census and counted 5,246 natives in the Marquesan Islands. There were 90,000 natives there around 1800. Much of the tattoo culture, which played a heavy part in the social structure of the conquered peoples, was lost.

Modern Christian conservatives continued the idea of tattoos as being for heathens. To this day, many religious conservatives still frown upon tattoos and other forms of body modification. In adapting to the evolving views of popular culture, the Catholic view on tattooing appears to be that it's okay as long as you get tattooed in a safe environment with as little risk to infection as possible. Catholicism also recommends that the tattoos be of good moral taste and not offend or cause harm to your fellow human beings.

Sailors were known for coming into port and spending all their money on booze and tattoos while causing a ruckus. This kept the old attitude that tattoos were for the barbaric alive and well. After being confined to a ship for an extended period of time and without much of anything to spend their money on, sailors would come into port for only a few nights looking for something to do. Due to a tradition of taking souvenirs and not particularly being held back by the attitudes of mainstream society, getting tattooed became a popular form of entertainment. It was, after all, the sailors who ventured to Polynesia and brought back with them the tribal tattoos as well as a means to create them. Like these sailors, for many people there is excitement in traveling and getting a tattoo. For this reason, some of the busiest tattoo shops today are the shops located in tourist destinations.

After WWII, many soldiers came home with tattoos they had gotten when overseas. Some of those soldiers rode motorcycles during the war and continued to do so when they returned to the United States. Anyone who rides a motorcycle can tell you it's fun to ride with friends. This enjoyment of riding with friends is what led to the formation of biker gangs. Thanks to *The Wild One* (1953) with Marlon Brando, which portrayed motorcycle gangs as rebellious and unruly, the motorcycle became a symbol of rebellion. Tattoos had been a sign of rebellion for years, so the two forms of rebellion became intertwined.

Not Just for Bikers Anymore

In the last two decades of the twentieth century, tattooing slowly gained popularity. The old association of tattoos and degenerates still existed, but more people wanted to get tattooed just to decorate their bodies instead of for showing a sign of rebellion. The start of custom tattoo shops also helped to bring more of a fine-art feeling to tattooing. Instead of just getting a random design off the wall, many people wanted to have a design made only for them. Slowly we are coming to terms with tattooing being more of an art form than a crude craft.

Tattoos are fun.

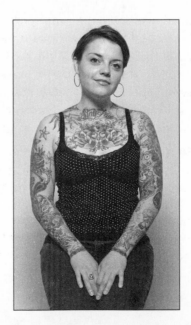

The idea of getting a tattoo as a souvenir is also becoming more popular as the tourism industry expands. People have more money and even more credit available than they did decades ago, which allows for more travel and more souvenirs. Many people today see getting a little tattoo as the equivalent to buying a new pair of shoes. A tattoo is just another thing one can purchase for fun.

With the advent of tattoo suppliers, more people have been able to break into tattooing as a profession. More shops have been opening, making it easier for people to get tattoos. Much of the old negative attitudes about tattooing are passing away with the older generations. Younger people are more used to tattoos, because they see them on their peers more often in public and especially on television, the Internet, and movies.

Professional athletes seem to be covered in tattoos nowadays. It used to be the stereotype that rock stars had tattoos. Now, sports associations such as the NBA are full of heavily tattooed players. Many boxers and Ultimate Fighters also sport tattoos in the ring. The more people of stature are seen with tattoos, the more open mainstream society becomes toward tattoos.

Rite of Passage

Tattooing has long been a way to mark a significant point in a person's life. Many tribal cultures use tattooing as a ritual to express the transformation of a child into an adult at the time of puberty. The reaction of the individual during the tattooing process will reveal his or her position in the tribe. If the adolescent quits or complains during the tattooing, it can lead to a low social position, especially if he is a chief's son.

Tattooing in the Western world is a little different now. A tattoo won't necessarily determine your place in the village, but it will show that you have become a legal adult. It may be a small celebration, but the significance of coming of age is great.

As we shall see later in this chapter, joining a gang or some form of club may require a tattoo to show the individual's commitment.

It is a permanent display of that group's ideology. It can mean a show of support and loyalty to the group, which will be seen by all the people in that person's everyday life.

Tattoos in the Workplace

Suits are great for covering tattoos. You may be surprised as to how many people are covering large tattoos under their long-sleeve shirts. Many people make sure their tattoos can be covered with a short-sleeve shirt to keep the boss from seeing it. Despite the wide acceptance of tattoos, it is still possible that a visible tattoo can keep one from getting a job. Employers sometimes still think a tattoo is a sign of rebelling, so think about the placement of your tattoo before you get it.

Becoming Heavily Tattooed

Becoming heavily tattooed means tattoos become a part of your life, like a hobby or a collection. There is a whole world out there of tattoos and tattoo paraphernalia. The Internet is loaded with tattoo-related blogs and chat rooms. There is a camaraderie that exists between heavily tattooed people.

Photo of a heavily tattooed person.

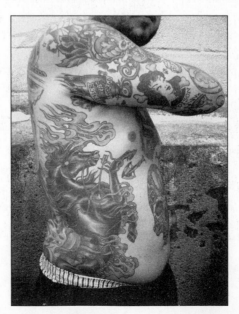

When you start to have visible tattoos, you will find that people treat you a little differently. People might stare at you more. Many people will talk to you about your tattoos and even try to touch you. It sounds freaky, but it's true. If you are polite about it, people will often be very polite back to you.

In some circumstances, you may find that people are more timid and stand-offish. This usually happens in small-town situations where there isn't a local tattoo shop and the attitudes toward tattoos haven't evolved. In the end, if you want to be heavily tattooed, it's your choice, and what other people think shouldn't matter.

Job Stoppers

A "job stopper" is a tattoo that is below the wrist or above the collarbone. These tattoos can make it very difficult to get a job despite the wide acceptance of tattoos. It is prohibited in many states and certain countries to tattoo someone below the wrist or on the neck or face.

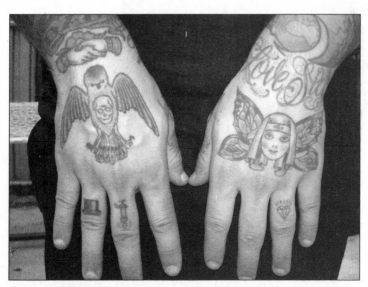

Tattooed hands by Dan Trocchio.

Some people want their first tattoo to be on their hand or neck. They think it looks pretty or will make them look tough. Tattooists will often tell these people about the consequences of such tattoos and try to persuade them to get the tattoo on a more discreet place. However, it is not the job of the tattooists to morally instruct clients.

If someone is bound and determined to get a job stopper, most tattooists are willing to oblige. It's best, though, to think about the consequences before you break the job-stopper barrier.

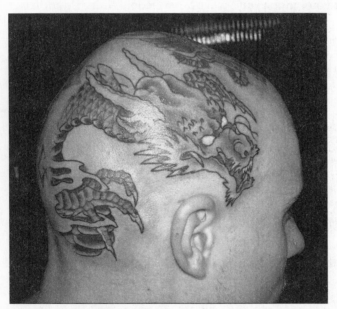

Wes Nile of the band Razorblade Hand Grenade; a tattoo by John Reardon.

Due to the wider acceptance of tattoos, it is hard to be considered rebellious unless you go that extra step to be an outsider. Going to extremes means having to push one step further. Most people who have hand and face tattoos get them because they think it's beautiful and they like the reaction, good or bad, that they get from other people, sometimes to the point of addiction.

Perhaps a feeling of already being an outcast pushes these people to further separate themselves from mainstream society. A sense of independence and freedom from the unwritten laws of social etiquette could be realized through the tattoo. Job stoppers are public statements that this individual shuns conformity. Whatever the individual's reasons for adorning him- or herself with nonconcealable tattoos, in the end, doing so shows a sign of commitment to the entity of tattooing.

Military Regulations

In order to keep the U.S. military looking professional, a few regulations on tattoos had to be put in place. These rules are pretty much the same for each branch as far as content and placement.

- ◆ **Navy**—Tattoos are not allowed on the head, face, neck, or scalp.

- ◆ **Army**—Tattoos are permitted on the hand and the back of the neck, but not on the front or side of the neck, or on the head or face. Permanent makeup is allowed on women but nothing too flashy.

- ◆ **U.S. Coast Guard**—Only 25 percent coverage is allowed on the arm between the wrist and elbow and on the leg between the knee and ankle. No tattoos are allowed on the hands, head, or neck.

- ◆ **Marines**—No tattoos are allowed below the elbow or below the knee. This is a new regulation, which started on April 1, 2007. Marines who already have tattoos on their forearms and legs aren't allowed to add on to them. The hands, neck, and head are also off-limits for tattoos.

- ◆ **Air Force**—Only one quarter of the exposed body part may be tattooed. Tattoos are not allowed above the collarbone or to be readily visible when wearing an open-collar uniform.

Keep in mind that in the military tattoo designs must be in good taste and cannot be gang related, indecent, extremist, sexist, or racist. The tattoos also cannot show poor morale.

Tattoo Taboo

If you are planning to join the military, be sure to ask a recruiter about the regulations of tattooing before you get tattooed, just to be safe.

Naval personnel have a long-running reputation of having tattoos. This, of course, comes from the old days of tattoo shops in ports and harbors. Many of the older designs from the '30s and '40s featured a pin-up girl in a sailor's uniform. Marines are also known to get marine-pride tattoos such as the USMC Bulldog.

Military flash design by Sam Hambrick.

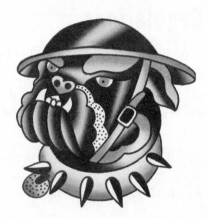

Gang Tattoos

As we have seen, tattoos have traditionally been associated with criminals in many societies. It is true that many gangs represent themselves with tattoos. The markings show the permanence of each member's dedication to the group as well as warning others to beware. Different parts of the world have developed different gangs.

In the twentieth century, we saw the rise of biker gangs such as the Hells Angels. The Hells Angels are now a motorcycle club and have a website and merchandise. They are known for having many tattoos and are involved with the security for many tattoo conventions as well as concerts. The Big Red Machine, as they are known, have chapters throughout the United States and throughout the world. Their famous logo is called the Deathshead, which is the profile of a skull with wings. The Hells Angels and other motorcycle clubs are very involved in the tattoo industry, and many members are often tattooists or shop owners.

Street gang members also are often tattoo collectors. Many will have the logo of the gang tattooed on themselves. It became so common for gang memberss to get gang-related tattoos that law officials have been studying the designs for years. Many police officials study these designs so that they can determine who is involved with whom. This is especially important for corrections officers, as many gang members are incarcerated. The violence is so bad that gangs are separated in jail.

Gangs are generally race oriented, which, in turn, determines the designs of gang tattoos. White power gangs often have Celtic or Viking designs. Designs from Northern Europe or Nazi Germany, which depict a cultural origin, are used to

> **Tattoo Taboo**
>
> It is not a good idea to get a gang- or club-related tattoo if you are not a member. The offended gang or club will likely remove the tattoo, or worse.

represent the various white supremacist groups such as the Aryan Brotherhood. Whites are a minority in the prison system and don't necessarily have a home turf or neighborhood like African Americans and Hispanics or Latinos.

Hispanic or Latino gangs tend to have tattoos with Christian themes such as crosses or praying hands. They also have developed a particular style of tattooing from their culture. They often have a Latino pin-up girl wearing a Stetson or fedora hat tattooed in a thin-line style and in black and gray. Jack Rudy, a tattooist from California, made these tattoo designs popular. Now Mr. Cartoon has made that style more popular by tattooing many hip-hop artists such as Eminem.

In the California correctional system, a group of Mexican Americans came together to create one of California's most notorious gangs, the Mexican Mafia. This group split in two to create the Surenos (southerners) and the Nortenos (northerners). The Surenos usually have tattoos with the letter 13, which can represent the letter M, as it is the thirteenth letter in the alphabet. La Ema, which is Spanish for M, shows respect to the Mexican Mafia. The Nortenos, who broke away from the Mexican Mafia in the late '60s, are based in Northern California. Both Latino gangs get tattoos to represent where they are from, such as an area code. They will also get a teardrop by the outside corner of their eyes to represent a murder committed or, more recently, to represent a fallen friend while they were in prison.

Inkformation

A popular tattoo in prison is 13½. This means 12 jurors, a judge, and a half-wit lawyer or half a chance.

Another Latino gang that is growing immensely in size is the gang known as MS-13. MS stands for Mara Salvatrucha. Mara refers to an army ant, while Salvatrucha is Spanish slang for Salvadorian. The group generally consists of Salvadorians but has been reported to include other Central Americans as well. The members will have MS-13 tattooed on them, or they might have a tattoo of devil horns, as the group took the horns hand gesture from early rock and metal shows. Many also have been seen with facial tattoos.

Gang style flash.

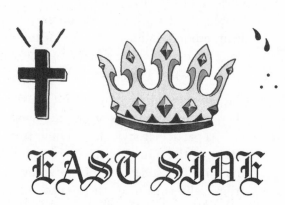

Most gang members will get words tattooed on them, which represent their gangs and where they are from. Old English is the most popular lettering used for all gangs. Many of the Latino gangs will use a very beautiful and decorative script. This form of lettering is very popular among tattooists. Good script is a sign of a good tattooist.

During the regime of the Soviet Union, a very complex, symbolic form of tattooing came about in the Russian prison system. As in most prisons, the ink was made from burning the heel of a shoe and then mixing it with urine to liquefy the dark soot. Many symbols have been created to show a person's rank in the prison and even to show if that person had screwed up. Grins are tattoos forced on prisoners who don't pay their gambling debts or who mess up in other ways. The image is usually of a sexual nature meant to be embarrassing for the wearer.

Inkformation

In Great Britain, prisoners would tattoo ACAB on their knuckles. It is an acronym for "All Cops Are Bastards" or "Always Carry a Bible," depending on whom the inmate was talking to.

Here are other symbols:

Spade: A thief.

Club: A criminal.

Diamond: A stool pigeon, a mark that is placed by force.

Heart: Sex symbol and a passive homosexual or a prison sex object.

Barbwire: The number of barbs in the wire shows how many years in the sentence.

Butterfly: Shows a trustworthy individual or an escape artist.

Crown: A king or head of a family.

Dagger with blood: A killer or one who will help with a murder.

Tattooing in North American prisons is illegal. Being caught can lead to a loss of privileges or of parole. There is no way of sanitizing anything and many diseases may have been transferred through prison tattooing. In Canada, where 26 percent of all inmates leave with fatal incurable diseases, a program is being set up where professional tattoo shops will be placed in prisons. They will be up to health-code standards and staffed by prisoners. This will enable prisoners to learn about a profession as well as get clean tattoos.

The Least You Need to Know

◆ Tattooing is slowly becoming more accepted in modern society.

◆ Becoming heavily tattooed will change your life.

◆ Face and hand tattoos can make it difficult to get a regular job.

◆ The military has restrictions about its soldiers getting tattooed.

◆ Tattoos serve as insignia for gangs and other social-fringe groups.

3

Different Styles of Tattooing

In This Chapter

- ◆ Different styles of lettering
- ◆ Most predominant styles
- ◆ Popular quickies
- ◆ Creating your own

For the first 100 years of modern tattooing, not too many significant innovations in tattoo design occurred. Not to say that there weren't any—there were—but due to the low number of tattooists working and the lack of communication between them, it was difficult for any form of group brainstorming to develop. Tattooists became very secretive and very competitive. Sharing secrets was unheard of.

With the connections of correspondences between tattooists such as Sailor Jerry Collins, Mike Malone, Kazuo Oguri, and Ed Hardy, the silence began to talk. More connections and friendships began to be made. Tattoo conventions opened things up even further. Tattooists from Europe and America started to work together more often. The '70s saw a new era of tattoo design innovation. The more people began to tattoo from different artistic backgrounds such as comic books or graffiti in the late '80s, the more different styles of tattooing began to appear.

Tattooists sold their designs to other tattooists, which further spread different concepts. More and more new ideas were available for reference. With the Internet, the spread of ideas and concepts became instantaneous with thousands of designs on the web. Individual tattooists could show what they were doing, which many times was something new outside the boundaries of a label.

What Is Flash?

In order for a tattoo shop to get as many tattoos done as possible per day, it needs to have tattoo designs ready to go. People who want to get tattooed also need a variety of designs to choose from. This is where flash comes in. Flash is the collection of designs for tattoos in a tattoo shop. Any design that is made so that many people can get it tattooed is considered flash.

Flash, in the United States, is traditionally printed on 14" × 11" pieces of paper. These pieces of paper are displayed throughout the tattoo shop so you will have a variety of designs to choose from. You can also use the designs to get an idea of what you want to have tattooed, as flash can be used for really good reference material.

As previously stated, having flash designs enables a tattooist to do many tattoos in one day. Just using flash keeps the tattooist from having to draw each tattoo from scratch, which can take hours to do. Many different people choose the same design over and over. It is not uncommon for a tattooist working in a street shop to do the same design more than twice in one day. The whole tattoo process is faster with flash, so you won't have to wait around as long. Also, if you choose a flash design, you can basically see beforehand what the tattoo will look like when it's done.

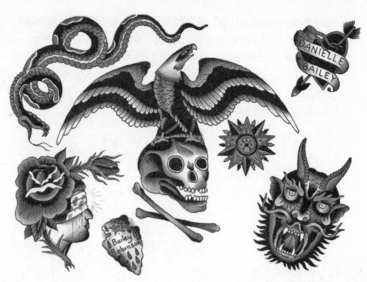

Traditional sheet of flash by Bailey Robinson. This is a traditional 14" × 11" sheet of flash that you will find in most shops.

Lettering

Lettering is very important in the tattoo business. There are so many reasons why people get lettering tattooed on them. It can be the most direct and obvious way to express yourself. Often lettering is used as a memorial of a lost loved one such as a relative or friend. Lettering is often used to show a person's past, origin, or group affiliation such as with a gang (as we learned in Chapter 2).

In many tattoo designs, lettering is used to enhance the design. Many people will actually base the image from a quote or a popular saying, such as "Born to Lose" or "Love Thy Neighbor." Lyrics from songs as well as text from the Bible are often used in tattoos.

Lettering can be very decorative, large, and creative or it can be small, plain, and basic. It all depends on personal taste or just what you want to say. Let's take a look at the different kinds of lettering most often used or asked for in tattooing.

Tattoo by John Reardon, 2004.

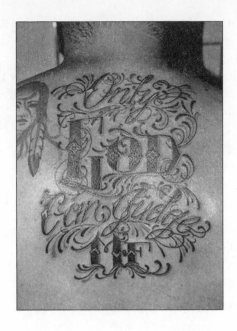

Script

Script lettering, or cursive handwriting, is one of the most popular lettering used in tattooing. It can be quick and simple or highly decorative. Many people will get their name or a name of a loved one in script, as it can be quick and not so expensive depending on the amount of detail. A word written in a good script can really enhance a tattoo design by making it more decorative and intricate.

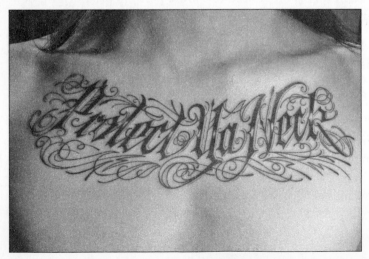

An example of script lettering. Tattoo by Joseph Ari Aloi (JK5)

Historically, script lettering was developed and came to popularity in the seventeenth and eighteenth centuries. It was created because there was a need for a faster form of legible standardized writing. Writing a word in one single stroke is much faster than printing each individual letter. One example of script can be seen in the American Declaration of Independence. The advent of the typewriter and then the computer has taken away the importance of script, leaving it to be more of an art form than a way of communication.

Script is now a necessary tool in the tattooist's arsenal. The skill of good script lettering is necessary in being a great tattooist. Many tattooists will practice script for hours to make sure they get it right.

Flash Tip

Script writing looks best when it is written horizontally from left to right. It doesn't work well written vertically.

Old English

Old English is actually a language and not a form of lettering. Blackletter is the actual term for what we think of as "Old English" lettering. Blackletter was created around 1150 C.E. and used until 1500 C.E. Old English the language was pretty much out of use by 1150 C.E. The Old English language was originally written with a runic alphabet before the introduction of the Latin alphabet around 600 A.D.

Just as script was used to improve the efficiency of handwriting, Blackletter was created to replace Carolingian Minuscule, which was used to reproduce religious texts. As more and more secular books needed to be reproduced, and all books were made by hand in this era because it was before the invention of the printing press, a faster and more modern lettering was needed. Blackletter was the answer. Its popularity ended in the sixteenth century with the exception of Germany, where it was used up until the twentieth century. It was then relabeled "Gothic Script," Gothic meaning barbaric, by Renaissance Humanists who thought the lettering was old-fashioned and out of style, linked to the medieval period.

Other than script, Old English lettering is the most-used form of lettering in the tattoo industry. It is very bold yet slightly decorative. As we learned in Chapter 2, Old English lettering is used for tattoo designs by almost every gang around. The popularity of it in mainstream America was broadened by the various bands and rap groups who had the lettering tattooed on them. Before that, it was popular with rockers, who preferred large lettering across the stomach or across the upper back. The smallest you can go with Old English lettering is about three quarters of an inch. If you want the lettering smaller, better to go with a simpler form of lettering.

Old English lettering.

OLD ENGLISH

Old English

Graffiti

Modern graffiti started in Philadelphia and quickly moved to New York City in the late 1960s. JULIO 204 is credited with its beginning as the first writer; TAKI 183 was the center of an article in the New York Times in 1971. Since then, modern graffiti has expanded all over the world and has become intertwined with many different industries.

Modern graffiti lettering has become popular in tattooing in the last 15 years. Many graffiti artists have picked up the tattoo machine like MED or SEEN from the Bronx. Oftentimes, tattooists with a graffiti background are able to create the best lettering for tattooing in any style, whether it's script or graffiti. If you want to get a tattoo with graffiti-style lettering, go to a good graffiti artist-turned-tattooist or just have a graffiti artist draw it for you. Only someone who is trained in that style can execute it properly.

Inkformation

Some graffiti legends from New York City have become tattooists such as MED and SEEN, who both have opened up their own tattoo shops in the Bronx.

Computer Fonts

There are so many fonts out there to choose from. Some people just want something quick and fairly basic. Many shops will have a book of computer fonts to choose from and many people just get some form of computer font instead of something custom like script. Often Old English lettering is just printed from the computer.

Using a computer font is a very efficient way to get lettering tattooed. The tattooist can simply manipulate the lettering on a computer; if you want the lettering on a curve or printed vertically, it just takes a few clicks of a mouse. The size can also be changed very easily on the computer.

Small, Basic Lettering

Many people like to get very small tattoos. As we know, that is perfectly fine as long as the design is simple and not too small. For lettering to be small, it has to be very basic in order to be legible and not to turn into a blob in 10 years.

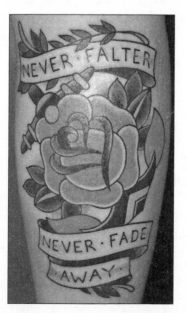

Simple lettering in a banner will make it easier to read. Tattoo by Steve Byrne.

Many tattoo designs have banners in them, which are used as space for lettering. Many times the banners will be too small for any fancy lettering such as script to fit inside them legibly. This is when you will want to use basic lettering. It will look much better and will be easier to read than trying to cram fancy lettering into a design.

Traditional Thick and Thin

Traditional thick and thin lettering is standard in tattoos. It is bold, simple, and will age well. It also allows for some color to be added in the thick parts. This style of lettering can be found in many Sailor Jerry designs.

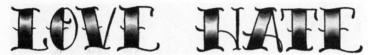

Traditional thick and thin lettering.

Traditional thick and thin lettering can be tattooed relatively small, making it good for banners. It is a little fancier than basic lettering so it can add some decoration to your tattoo without becoming overbearing. It is often used for finger tattoos due to its bold simplicity.

Drop Shadows

Drop shadows are lines or shading added to lettering to make the lettering a little more decorative. A shadow or line is placed next to the lettering, usually down and to the right, to make it appear more three-dimensional or just to make the lettering more dynamic. Drop shadows can be in any direction or even be done to a one-point perspective (when the perspective comes from one fixed position). It's all a matter of personal taste. They can be done in black or color, but are usually done in gray.

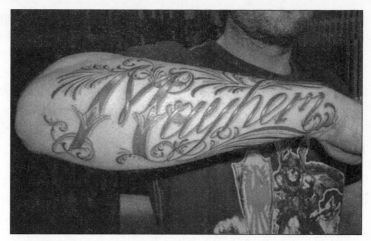

An example of a script tattoo that uses a thin line down and to the right as a drop shadow. Tattoo by John Reardon.

Other Languages

It is very popular to have a tattoo done in a language that is not based on the English alphabet. Words written in Chinese or Japanese are popular tattoos. The classical Indian language of Sanskrit is popular as well. These are all well and good to have tattooed, but you must remember that most tattooists do not understand how these languages are written or put together. They may not know how to correctly calligraph the design if it is not already calligraphied. If you want to get a foreign language tattooed, come with the design prepared so it won't be tattooed incorrectly.

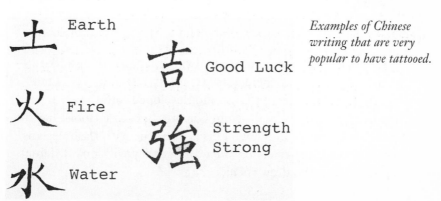

土 Earth

吉 Good Luck

強 Strength
   Strong

火 Fire

水 Water

Examples of Chinese writing that are very popular to have tattooed.

Many shops will have some words in a foreign language ready to go. If they don't have what you are looking for, you can always go to a restaurant advertising the country whose language you want tattooed and ask them to write the word or phrase out for you. Just make sure they do it cleanly and calligraph it for you, or else it won't work. If it is possible, go to a different restaurant advertising the same country and ask them to read it back to you to make sure you haven't been tricked.

> ### Tat-tale
>
> In a tattoo shop, not too far away, a large man was having his name, written in Japanese, tattooed on his neck. The man had decided to bully a reluctant Japanese waiter at a nearby restaurant into writing the name on a piece of paper. Unbeknownst to the bully, the waiter did not translate the name, but wrote "big stupid oaf" in Japanese.

The Internet has many translating websites that make getting a foreign-language tattoo much easier. Be aware, with Chinese and Japanese, putting certain characters next to each other may change the meaning. Also, if you want to get your name tattooed in a foreign language, it may not be possible. Remember that most people in China aren't named Charlie or Vanessa. Your name will not exist in their language. You must also remember that their language is not based on the ABCs, so you can't have your name spelled out. It just isn't possible. The Japanese language does have a set of characters designed for foreign languages. You may be able to have your name written in that.

Images

Most tattoos will consist of some form, image, or design like a tiger or a rose. Many themes are repeated over and over. They are translated by each tattooist and developed into something new over time. As we will see in Chapter 8, each tattooist has his or her own style of drawing. This is also true with flash designs. You may see many tigers on the wall but they will look different, depending on who drew them.

There are a few basic styles that have developed over the years to become the staples of what you will find in the flash racks. These are major styles that have become most popular. Let's go over them so you will know what you are looking at as you search through the flash for your design.

Tribal

As we learned in Chapter 1, tribal tattooing is mainly based on designs from the South Pacific. There are many tattooists who carry on the tradition today and still tattoo the original designs or very similar variations of them. It was Leo Zulueta who pioneered modern tribal tattoo designs in the early 1980s in California. Most of the tribal designs you see in tattoo shops come from Leo Zulueta's innovations.

Tribal is generally tattooed with all-black ink, which makes it great for the aging process. You can have color or gray incorporated into the design depending on personal taste. When looking for a good tribal design, it is important to remember that the negative space around the design is as important as the tattooed part of the design. It's the balance or play between the two that makes for a good tribal design.

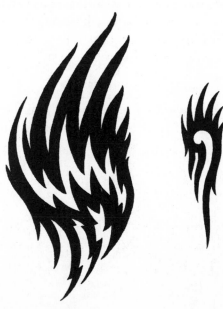

A few basic examples of modern tribal designs.

With most modern tribal tattoos, you must realize that there is no meaning to them and that they are just designs. You can always have a custom tribal design drawn that will have meaning to you, but there is no hidden language to speak of. Some designs may be in the shape of an animal or mythological beast like a shark or a dragon. Some of the most popular tattoo designs are a tribal armband or a tribal tattoo placed on the lower back of a woman.

Portraits/Realistic

Portraits and realistic tattooing can be one of the most difficult styles to tattoo. A tattooist must be very good at drawing and be very experienced with the medium to do this kind of tattooing. If you want to get a tattoo like this, find an expert or you may end up with an unfixable mess.

When getting a portrait-style tattoo of a loved one, such as a family member, there are a few things you will need, and need to know.

1. Bring a very clear photograph, preferably professionally done. Snapshots may not work and Polaroids are out of the question.

2. To get the correct amount of detail, the face must be around 3 inches, if not larger, when tattooed. Some very skilled tattooists can do it a little smaller.

3. The tattoo will look like the photo. Use a photo that is characteristic of the person you want a tattoo of.

4. Using black and gray is the easiest way to have the portrait tattooed but some tattooists can do an amazing job in color.

For realistic tattoos of subjects other than someone you know personally, like a musician, character in a movie, or some kind of animal, the same rules apply as with portraits. Usually you will be able to find the photo or image you are looking for on the Internet. Magazines such as *Rolling Stone* or *National Geographic* are good sources also. Just remember, the tattoo will look like the image you bring to the tattooist.

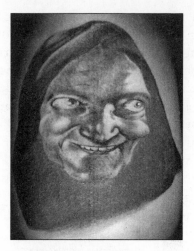

Realistic tattoo. Tattoo by Miss D'Joe, Lark Tattoo, Westbury, NY, www.larktattoo.com.

Biomechanical

Biomechanical tattoos are based on the artistic style of H. R. Giger. An example of this style can be seen in the design of the movie series *Alien*. The style combines organic and natural design with industrial design. It was Aaron Cain who made the style popular with tattooing in the 1990s. Biomechanical is a good design style for covering old tattoos. There is a lot of detail, which will help camouflage the older tattoo, and it is a style that can be quite dark and still look good.

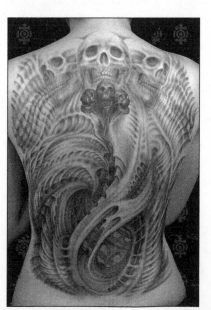

Biomechanical tattoo by Matthew Amey, www.independenttattoo.com.

Traditional

Traditional tattooing was originally developed by the sailors who brought back tattooing from the South Pacific. It is characterized as having thick bold lines, plenty of black shading, stiff or static drawing, and a very simplified and flat appearance. Often the designs will have few colors, usually consisting of red, yellow, orange, and olive green. Traditional tattoos are very good at standing the test of time. Sailor Jerry Collins was known for his style and is a huge influence on traditional tattooists today.

Traditional tattoo by Bert Krak, Top Shelf Tattoo, Bayside, NY, www. bertkrak.com.

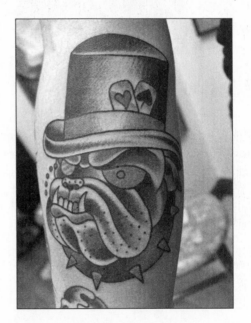

Traditional tattoos have had a huge revival in the last decade. Many tattooists specialize in this style. They use designs from the early twentieth century. A good example of this can be seen in the book *Revisited: A Tribute to Flash from the Past* by Steve Boltz and Bert Krak. In the book, different tattooists from around the world redrew old flash from the early twentieth century.

New School

The New School style came into existence around the end of the 1980s and the beginning of the 1990s from tattooists like Marcus

Pacheco. New School tattoo designs combine traditional and Japanese themes with a modern graffiti style. They allow for more dimensional shading with the use of one or more light sources. The lines of New School tattoos will often be calligraphied. The style allows for very bright colors and animated drawings.

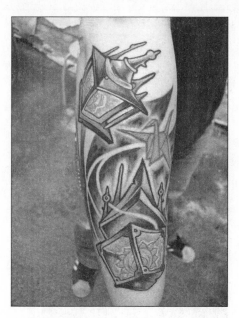

New school tattoo by Brian Awake.

Japanese

Japanese-style tattoos have been around for over 200 years. They are characterized by relatively large images of Japanese folklore or traditions in the foreground, such as a *hanya mask* or a dragon surrounded by a stylized black and gray background of clouds or water. The designs are elegant, and they fit to the body well. One Japanese tattoo style, which is called a body suit, can cover your entire body. Only a master of this style such as Horiyoshi III or Horitoshi will be able to create tattoos of this caliber.

Today, many tattooists from around the world work in this style such as Filip Leu and Alex Reinke. It takes many years to learn the style of Japanese tattooing and requires a study of Japanese culture. Many tattooists combine the Japanese style with other elements or themes of tattooing.

Inkformation _____

A **hanya mask** is a mask used in traditional Japanese Noh theater. It is characterized by having two pointed horns and sharp teeth much like a western devil. The image can also be used to scare off evil spirits by hanging a mask on a wall in your house or having it tattooed on your

Japanese style tattoo by Mike Rubendall, www.kingsavenuetattoo.com.

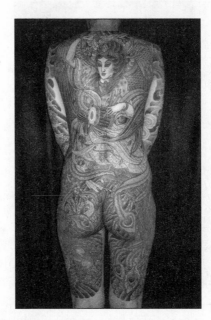

Fine-Line Black and Gray

Fine-line black and gray tattooing became very popular in the 1970s in Southern California. The style uses thin lines made with a single pin needle or a three-pin needle, and has very smooth and dimensional black and gray shading. The designs are often accompanied with fancy script-style lettering. Often religious themes such as a sacred heart or the Virgin Mary will be used. Tattooist Jack Rudy, who has been seen tattooing Jesse James on *Monster Garage*, is one of the artists who made innovations in this style and helped to popularize it in the late 1970s.

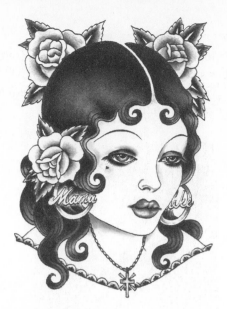

An example of fine line black and gray flash. Tattoo by Katja Ramirez, Houston, TX, www.kotattoos.com.

Quick Little Ones

Most people are happy with little tattoos. Often tattoo shops located in or near a tourist destination will be bombarded with people who just want small little collectables. There are a few designs that seem to be the most popular for this situation. Let's take a look at what they are and what they mean.

The Nautical Star

A very popular tattoo is the nautical star. It hails from the days of the sailor. Sailors would get them tattooed as good-luck charms. They stand as a symbol of protection and guidance. Today, many rock bands will use this symbol or have it tattooed. This symbol is also often used as decoration for tattoos that are sea-related such as a sailing ship or a rock of ages.

A nautical star.

The Rose

Roses are extremely popular in tattooing. They are often used to decorate other themes such as the Virgin of Guadalupe. A small rose is a symbol of love and romance. Many times the name of a lover will be tattooed with a small rose.

A simple rose design by John Reardon.

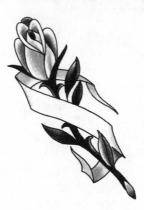

The Butterfly

Butterflies are popular tattoos for women to get and sometimes for men, too. The design allows for lots of bright colors and can be added to later with flowers or more butterflies. Butterflies are a symbol of change, as they change from a not-so-attractive caterpillar into a beautiful butterfly. They are also a symbol of joy.

A traditional butterfly design by John Reardon.

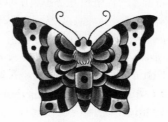

Looking for Something Specific

If you are looking for something more specific, like a particular animal in a certain pose that you can't find in the tattoo shop, look online or at the library. Google will have lots of photos to choose from. Dover publishing (www.doverpublishing.com) publishes books on everything that makes great tattoo designs. You don't have to be restricted by the flash on the wall. You can find a design for a tattoo anywhere.

Large Custom Tattoos

Large custom tattoos, like a back piece or a sleeve, can be of any subject or theme. You can use flash designs for reference or even as the entire piece, but most tattooists, if putting so much energy into such a large piece, will want to customize the tattoo. It will make the process more personal for both of you, and you will have an original tattoo that no one else shares.

When looking for ideas for a large tattoo, it is best to start looking through portfolios with custom tattoos so you can see what can be done. You may see the idea you are looking for. Many people like to get traditional tattoo ideas like a dragon or a battle royal. A battle royal is a battle between an eagle, snake, and a dragon usually done in a traditional tattoo style.

One of the best ways to find an idea that most suits you is to think of all the stuff that you are into, like cars or antiques. What are your hobbies? What do you collect? What do you do on the weekends? Has there been a moment that has changed your life that you want to remember? Is there someone who has influenced you such as a historical figure? Research these ideas and events at the library or on the Internet. Put together a folder of reference material and maybe a little synopsis so that the tattooist can have a good idea of what you want. Your tattooist will guide you as to what works best and will shoot some ideas at you to make it better. Often he can explain how to decorate the idea to give it better design. With the right references for your subject, a good tattooist can turn it into a great tattoo.

*Large custom tattoo example
by Mike Rubendall,
www.kingsavenuetattoo.com.*

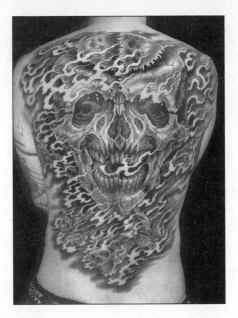

The Least You Need to Know

- There are many different kinds of fonts that you can use in tattooing.

- Script and Old English are the most popular fonts that people get tattooed.

- You will find a few basic styles in the flash racks in a tattoo shop.

- Some popular small tattoos are nautical stars, roses, and butterflies.

- You don't have to rely on flash for a tattoo; you can find a tattoo design anywhere.

4

The Science

In This Chapter

◆ What skin is made of

◆ How tattoos stay in the skin, and why they fade

◆ Tattooing techniques

◆ The pain factor

◆ Tattoo reactions

Now that we know the origins and social aspects of tattooing, we can move on to understanding how tattoos work. It is important to understand the details of how the ink stays in your skin and the different layers of your skin. This information will help you to properly care for your tattoo.

In this chapter, we will go over the fundamentals of tattooing, such as how tattoos stay in the skin and how they age. We will also go over the different pieces of the tattoo process as well as what to expect as far as pain. When it is your turn to get tattooed, you will understand more of what's going on and perhaps feel much more comfortable.

Your Skin

Skin is one of the most important organs of our bodies. It weighs more than any other organ, coming in at a whopping 15 percent of our body weight. Skin protects us by keeping disease from entering our bodies. Skin also protects us from the harmful rays of the sun. Most important, skin is where we keep our tattoos.

def•i•ni•tion

Skin is made up of three layers: the epidermis, the dermis, and the hypodermis.

Because your skin is the outermost layer of your body, it is what everyone sees. This seems like an obvious concept, but the importance of that fact has led to numerous multibillion-dollar industries. How much do people spend on skin products to keep themselves looking young? How often have you gone tanning? What brand of soap do you use? These all involve your outermost physical layer, your skin.

Layers of skin.

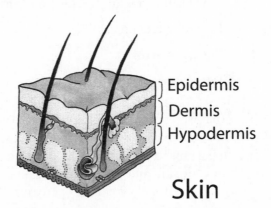

Epidermis
Dermis
Hypodermis

Skin

You probably studied the physical aspects of skin in some form of high school biology class. Just in case you weren't paying attention or simply forgot, let's go over the components of skin. Understanding your skin will help you to understand how a tattoo works.

Epidermis

The epidermis is the top layer of skin. It is the waterproof layer around your body. The waterproofing caused by keratin, a tough and insoluble protein. Carrots are a good source of keratin. As the cells of the epidermis move away from the body, they become cut off from the blood supply. Being removed from the blood source, the cells die and they are filled with keratin, making them stronger. This strong layer gives you more protection from disease.

The epidermis is also where *melanin* is produced. Melanin is the dark pigment in your skin made by melanocytes, which reside in the very first layer of your epidermis, directly above the dermis. Melanin rests above the other skin cells' nuclei in order to protect the DNA from the sun's ultraviolet light. The more melanin your skin produces, the darker your skin will be.

def•i•ni•tion

Melanin is a dark pigment made by your skin to protect your skin from the harmful rays of the sun.

Dermis

The dermis is the next layer of skin below the epidermis. It contains all the good, fun stuff, which gives your skin life. In the dermis are hair follicles, blood vessels, and sweat glands. It is also where the nerve endings are. The nerve endings enable us to feel sensations such as heat and cold and getting a tattoo. As we will find out, the dermis is also where the ink for the tattoo will stay.

Hypodermis

The hypodermis is the third layer, which is below the dermis. This layer is mainly for storing fat and holding some proteins. The thickness of the hypodermis depends on the amount of fat stored in the body.

How Tattoos Work

A tattoo is made by implanting *pigment* into the dermis, or second layer of skin. A tattoo is similar to a mini-implant. You are implanting tiny granules of color into your skin. Those tiny pieces of pigment are held in place by your skin's immune system. Your skin has cells called phagocytes. The phagocytes engulf the color particle, which then holds the color particle in place while your skin heals. When the tattoo is fully healed, the color particle will become trapped in place. It is trapped in the connective tissues just below the border between your epidermis, the first layer, and your dermis, the second layer.

def•i•ni•tion

Pigment is the colored powder material that is the base of inks used in tattoos.

Ink is implanted by a needle.

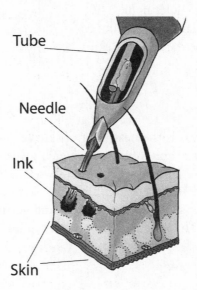

Tube

Needle

Ink

Skin

Because melanin is produced just above the dermis where the tattoo pigment will reside, the melanin will dilute or partially block the reflection of light from the tattoo pigment. This is why tattoo ink color is not as bright and is harder to see on darker skin.

The pigment of a recent tattoo is very easy to see because it is so close to the surface of the skin. You can see the pigment right through the first layer of skin. However, as time goes by and skin ages, the pigment slowly recedes more deeply into the dermis layer of the skin. This puts more tissue between the tattoo and the top layer, making the tattoo appear blurry and harder to see. This happens over decades, so no need to worry. Your tattoo will look great for a long time.

Inkformation

An accidental stabbing with a pen or pencil where the skin has been penetrated can permanently leave pigment in the skin like a tattoo.

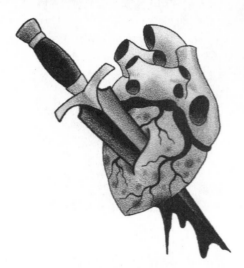

Standard flash design. Design by Eli Quinters, Brooklyn, NY, www. tattoosfortheunloved.com.

Various Techniques

As we learned in Chapter 1, tattooing developed at different times and in different ways throughout the world. Different techniques of putting pigment into the skin have emerged, as well as different designs. Some cultures created large ornamental tattoos while others were satisfied with smaller designs. Let's look at the different techniques that came about.

Hand Poked

Before the advent of electricity, all tattoos were done by hand. Different techniques of hand-poked tattooing have developed over the last 5,000 years. There are three different techniques that are the most popular today.

One technique, which can be found in prisons or in the hands of the less professional, is the single sewing-needle technique. All you need to perform this kind of tattoo is a (hopefully) sterile needle and some nontoxic, clean ink.

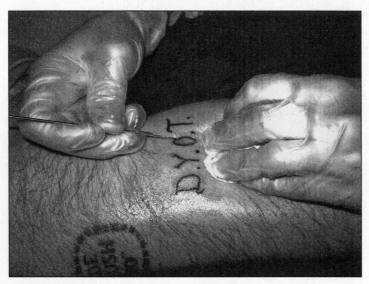

Hand-poked tattoo by Wes Nile.

One can put a little ink on the skin and poke away or use a thread wrapped near the tip of the needle to hold the ink. This technique is not the best and requires lots of time and patience for good results. In the right hands, however, fun and interesting tattoos can happen, which will mark an experience you will never forget.

def·i·ni·tion

Irizumi is the Japanese term for tattooing.

The second technique is a more developed version of the first. It's called *irizumi*, and it is from Japan. With irizumi, many needles are attached to the end of a rod made of either bamboo or stainless steel. The rod is usually no longer than a foot and a half. The tattooist dips the needle end of the rod into the ink cap and then pokes the skin rhythmically. In the right hands, this technique can be very fast and extremely solid and dense.

A similar technique is used in Thailand for religious and spiritual reasons. A priest or monk will use a long metal rod, which is pointed at one end. The pointed end is dipped in ink, then used to tattoo.

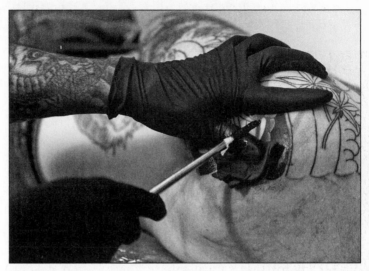

Traditional Japanese tattooing by Shinji.

The third technique comes form tribal tattooing in the Pacific. A stick with a sharpened bone or stick on the end of it, at a 90-degree angle, is held over the skin and then tapped into the skin with another stick. Nowadays, many traditional tribal tattooists will use a sterilized needle on the end of the tattooing stick. These tattoos are usually geometric in design and can be quite painful.

Machine Work

Most modern tattoos are done with an electric tattoo machine. If you walk into just about any tattoo shop in the world, the tattoo you get will be done with an electric tattoo machine. It is the most efficient way to do tattoos. Machine work is generally faster than tattoos done by hand, which enables tattooists to do many tattoos in one day.

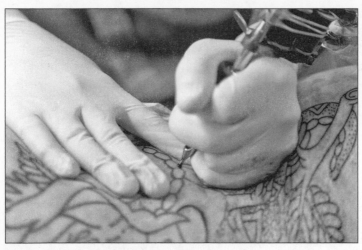

Modern method—tattooing in action.

The One-Point Tattoo

Most people will only get a one-point tattoo. A one-point tattoo is a tattoo that is usually done in one session and drawn from one vantage point. Usually first-time tattoos are one-point tattoos.

One-point tattoo by John Reardon.

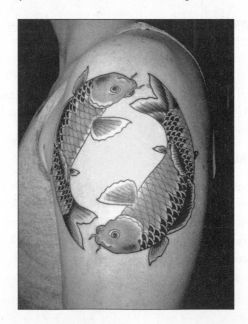

One-point tattoos are nice because you can have many of them from many different tattooists, like collecting stickers. They are also nice if you want to get tattoos to commemorate different times in your life. They are generally quick, so you don't have to come back again and again. There is less of a commitment with a one-point tattoo, and because of its smaller size, it can be easily hidden if you need it to be.

Serious Coverage

You can tell tattoo enthusiasts by the color of their skin, or better put, by the amount of colors in their skin. As tattooing is becoming more and more accepted by mainstream society, more people are getting large tattoos such as sleeves, a tattoo that covers the entire arm.

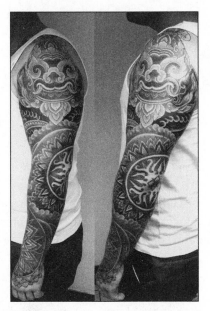

A full sleeve by Thomas Hooper, New York Adorned, New York, NY, www. nyadorned.com

To become heavily tattooed with large pieces, you must be prepared to commit yourself to getting your work completed. Large tattoos can cost as much as a car, but they will last much longer. Socially, large tattoos will change your life. You will almost always stick out in a crowd if you have many visible tattoos.

Yes, It Hurts

Pain is always a factor when getting a tattoo. It is inevitable to feel something while under the needle. Some people say they like the feeling of getting a tattoo. Some people don't seem to be affected by it too much. Luckily for us, there are easy spots on the body, which aren't as painful. However, some places are very sensitive. As a general rule, your first tattoo will be the easiest.

Most first-time tattoos are very small and take only 10 to 20 minutes, tops. That is a very short time-period to get tattooed. By the time you get used to the feeling, you are done. There is not even enough time to complain about it or take a break. The most painful spots can be easy to handle if the tattoo is small. It's the larger tattoos you want to worry about.

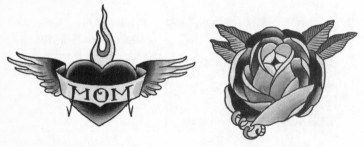

Flash of a small rose and heart.

There is more to endure with any tattoo that takes over an hour. With larger tattoos, placement is a factor. If you do not like pain at all, you will want to get your tattoo on a less painful place. It will be easier for you and the artist as well as being less dramatic.

The Easy Spots

There are a few spots on the body that are less painful to have tattooed. These places happen to be the most popular areas men have tattooed. They are the forearm and the outside of the upper arm. These are generally the easiest places to get tattooed. Every individual is different, and certain places may not hurt certain people as much as others. However, the arms and forearms, as a general rule, are the least painful places.

Everywhere Else

The rest of the body is fairly sensitive. Shoulder blades and certain spots on the legs aren't too painful. Any spot around a joint such as a wrist or the back of the knee can be extra sensitive. Hands and feet are quite uncomfortable to have tattooed. The ribs are known to be the worst place to get tattooed. This is not only because of sensitivity, but also because of the amount of space being tattooed. Generally, tattoo designs for the ribs are large in order to cover the entire area well. The front part of the torso is very sensitive.

The More You Get, the More It Hurts

If you want to be heavily tattooed, you will soon find that you have tattooed all the easy spots and have nothing but the less comfortable places left. Also you may not be the spring chicken you once were and now find that age has intensified the feeling of getting tattooed. All of these are factors in making tattooing more painful. Don't worry, though; you have to get a lot of tattoos before the notion of "the more you get, the more it hurts" comes into play.

Tat-tale

There once was a man who thought he was so tough, he could get a tattoo from his chest to his wrist, all in one session. In only one hour of tattooing, the "tough guy" couldn't take any more, so he paid the artist, ran out the door, and was never seen again.

Allergies

It is not uncommon to have some form of allergic reaction to a tattoo. Many people have a reaction to certain reds. Usually the affected area just swells or puffs up a bit and itches a little more than usual. That part of the tattoo may take a week or two longer to heal. On rare occasions, the red area in a tattoo will ooze a clear liquid called sebum. If that is the case, it is a good idea to tell the artist and find the name of that ink, so that you won't ever have it used on you again. It will be a few weeks before the tattoo heals, and it will be uncomfortable while it is healing.

Inkformation

Staph infection is an infection caused by spherical bacteria called *Staphylococcus aureus*. The bacteria can live on the skin or in the nose of a person and can be the cause of illnesses from skin infections and pimples to pneumonia and toxic shock syndrome.

Sometimes, the tattooed area breaks out in little pimples. This is usually a bad reaction to petroleum-based products, such as the lubrication used during the tattooing or the lotion you use afterward. Stop using the petroleum-based product and switch to a mild, unscented skin moisturizer. The pimples and itch should go away in a few days. If the area does not recover, then see a doctor because it may be a staph (bacterial) infection.

Scars

Scarring from a tattoo can happen to anyone. No matter how good the tattooist is, if you don't take good care of your tattoo, it can scar. An inexperienced tattooist is more likely to scar a client. This happens when the tattooist goes too deep or tattoos in one area, overworking and chewing the skin. Also, if you pick the scabs of your tattoo, you can damage your still-healing skin, which will leave a scar and possibly leave a blank spot in your tattoo.

Certain parts of the body are more prone to scarring. Skin that is near or on a joint is often tricky to tattoo and can scar easily. The skin over your iliac crest, or your hip bone, is often a tricky spot to tattoo. Your pants or skirt will rest on this area and will rub against the tattoo while you walk. This makes for a difficult healing process. Usually a piece of plastic wrap placed over the tattoo will block the friction of your clothes. If your tattoo scars a little, you can treat this by keeping it moist with vitamin

E oil, *A&D ointment*, or an unscented skin lotion supplemented with vitamins.

Many people want to have old scars covered up with tattoos. This is very possible, as we shall see in Chapter 6. Scars

def•i•ni•tion

A&D ointment is a petroleum-based product that contains vitamins A and D, and can be used to heal a tattoo as well as diaper rash.

are tricky to tattoo over. A scar occurs when the dermis layer of the skin is damaged. When the skin regenerates, the dermis can't reproduce itself complete with sweat glands, hair follicles, etc. Collagen, a strong fibrous protein, is made by the body to replace the lost dermis, leaving behind a smooth, discolored patch of skin. Because the melanocyte cells, the melanin-producing cells mentioned previously, may not be replaced, scar tissue is more susceptible to the harmful UV rays of the sun. Let's go over the different kinds of scars that are more common and find out how they occur.

Hypertrophic Scars

Hypertrophic scars are scars that heal a little puffy. They are raised up but not solid. With hypertrophic scars, the regenerating skin cells grow larger than they should. For all you weight lifters, this is similar to what happens to your muscles after training. You end up with larger muscles after an extended period of training. Hypertrophic scars can improve over time and don't grow beyond the original wound. A hypertrophic scar can be tattooed over if it has healed. Usually about 6 months to a year is a long enough healing time, but you should ask your doctor before tattooing over.

Keyloids

Keyloid scars occur when the collagen made to repair the abrasion grows out of control. A keyloid scar is firm and rubbery, and can grow into a benign tumor. The scar can itch or produce a needle-like pain. If scratched, the keyloid can get worse, which makes removing it surgically a problem. Over 50 percent of keyloid-removal surgeries result in another keyloid. This makes tattooing over a keyloid dangerous, and it should be avoided.

People with dark skin are more prone to keyloids, particularly people who are of African descent. Keyloids are used in many tribal cultures as a form of body modification and rites of passage. The skin is lacerated on certain parts of the body to create a puffy skin pattern. This is popular with the Nuba women in Sudan. The puffy keyloid scars depict the passages of life. Unfortunately, this may become extinct due to the atrocities occurring in that country.

Stretch Marks

Stretch marks are common, as any woman who has given birth or any person who has gained weight can tell you. Stretch marks usually occur around areas of the body that are prone to store fat, such as the stomach, breasts, thighs, hips, and buttocks. Anytime the skin is stretched beyond its normal capacity, such as during a pregnancy, stretch marks may develop. Many people try to cover stretch marks with tattoos, which works well in distracting the eye away from the scar, but the scar will still be there.

The skin develops stretch marks because glucocorticoid hormone, a form of steroid hormone, keeps the skin from producing collagen and elastin fibers, which are key to keeping skin firm as it grows rapidly. Unable to reproduce or grow fast enough, the dermis will split or crack, like the ground in an earthquake, due to a lack of support. Stretch marks won't form during body growth if there is enough support for the dermis.

A commonly asked question is whether a tattoo on the stomach will be ruined by stretch marks during pregnancy. This may deter women from getting a tattoo. It is true that stretch marks can run through a tattoo and disfigure the design. Disfigurement can occur anywhere on the body that you might get stretch marks while pregnant, not just on the stomach. It is possible to have the tattoo fixed or covered with another design.

Stretch marks during a pregnancy and the possible ruining of a tattoo can be avoided. Some women are more prone to the scars than others, but steps can be taken to lessen the effect. During pregnancy, if the woman has a strict daily routine of applying

Gotu Kola extract, vitamin E oil, and collagen hydrosolates, she can reduce the effects of stretch marks. Be sure you consult your doctor beforehand to make sure you won't have any reaction to the ingredients.

Giving Blood

After being poked with a tattoo needle, giving blood should be easy. At least you get a cookie for giving blood, not to mention that you could be saving someone's life. In the United States, most states will not allow you to give blood for one year after getting a tattoo. If you have a fear of hypodermic needles, then getting a tattoo is a good excuse to not give blood. However, if you get the tattoo in a tattoo shop that is licensed and state regulated, and the shop is eligible, you can get a voucher to give blood.

The Least You Need to Know

◆ Skin is made up of three layers: the epidermis, dermis, and hypodermis.

◆ Tattoo pigment is held in the skin by phagocytes in the upper layer of the dermis, just below the epidermis.

◆ There are different techniques for tattooing, but using a tattoo machine is by far the most common.

◆ Getting tattooed on most of the body can be quite painful, but small tattoos don't take too long, so it doesn't hurt as long.

◆ You can have an allergic reaction to a tattoo, but it is rare and easy to deal with.

◆ Most scars that have had time to heal can be tattooed over.

5

What Makes the Mark

In This Chapter

- ◆ How tattoo machines work
- ◆ What a tattoo needle looks like
- ◆ What equipment is used
- ◆ How the equipment is cleaned
- ◆ The basics of ink

Tattoo equipment is very sacred to a tattooist. The tools the tattooist uses determine how well the tattoo will turn out. It usually takes years for a tattooist to find the equipment that works the best. Learning how to adjust the equipment to work in just the right way takes lots of time and patience. Years of trying new and different techniques and equipment have led tattooists to be very secretive about the brand of tools and techniques they use.

In this chapter, you will get a glimpse of the equipment you will see when you get your tattoo. We will go over the basics of how tattoo machines work and the equipment needed to run them. This information is to help you relax when you get your tattoo by letting you get a little more familiar with the process. You may not want to have too many questions running through your head while you are waiting for your tattooist to start tattooing you. Having a good understanding of the equipment you see during your tattoo will make your experience much less intimidating. The more relaxed you are, the better.

The Tattoo Machines

The advent of the twentieth century brought in many new inventions and innovations to make people's lives much easier and more efficient. The widespread use of electricity brought with it many new inventions that were mass-produced and sold to the public. Western tattooing at this time was taken out of the dark ages: electricity was incorporated into the process of tattooing. This enabled tattoo artists to work with greater speed, and more customers were able to be tattooed in one day. The world of tattooing was becoming more of an industry. Early entrepreneurs started to make some real money from selling tattoo equipment and tattoo designs.

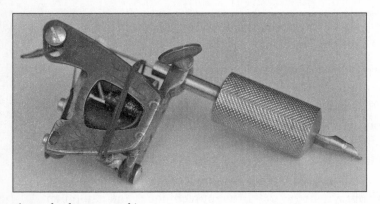

A standard tattoo machine.

Tattoo Taboo

A tattoo machine is called a "tattoo machine." It is a machine and there is no such thing as a tattoo "gun."

Most tattoos today are done with an electric tattoo machine. There are plenty of great artists who use the traditional methods (by hand) of tattooing; they keep the tradition alive and are sought out by tattoo enthusiasts. Many of these traditional tattooists can still tattoo with an electric machine if they need to. If you walk into any tattoo shop in the world, chances are you will be tattooed with a tattoo machine. It's much faster and more efficient for small designs.

The Creators

New York City takes the credit for being the birthplace for the first electric tattoo machine. It was in 1891, when a man by the name of Samuel O'Reilly patented the first electric tattoo machine. Samuel O'Reilly opened his first tattoo shop in 1875. It was located in Chatham Square, which is in what is now Chinatown, by the Manhattan entrance to the Manhattan Bridge. O'Reilly took an electric engraving device, which was invented by Thomas Edison, and modified it to be able to tattoo. This device was based on a rotary system. The needle was attached to a circular spinning device to make it go up and down. O'Reilly could now tattoo faster than anyone else in the world.

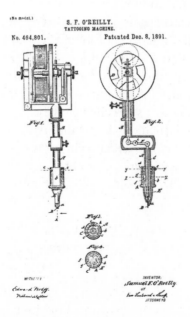

The O'Reilly patented machine.

(Photo courtesy of Tattoo Archive)

Seeing the upper hand that the rotary machine gave him, O'Reilly quickly offered the device for sale along with colors and designs. This paved the way for many people to become tattooists. Tattoo shops began to spring up throughout the major cities and also set O'Reilly up with a small fortune. Many other tattoo supply companies began to sell similar machines and equipment. More and more tattoo studios opened and the industry flourished.

Most modern tattoo machines aren't based on O'Reilly's rotary design. Today's machines are based on electromagnetic coils, although some people still use rotary machines. Thomas Riley of London had the first coil tattoo machine patent, which he got in 1891. This patent is closer to modern-day tattoo machines.

Over time the electric tattoo machine was tuned and perfected. Tattooists began to develop techniques to make the machine run better. A well-run and well-tuned machine is imperative in making a great tattoo. It will cause less damage to the skin, so the tattoo will heal quickly and look like it did when you left the tattoo shop.

How Modern Tattoo Machines Work

The modern tattoo machine is a very simple device. It is a two-coil electromagnet, which turns itself on and off through the breaking of its own circuit, like a doorbell. Electricity is fed to the machine by a clip cord via a power supply, which we will go over later in the chapter. The electricity magnifies the electromagnetic coils and pulls a small metal bar, called an armature bar, down to the coils. The end of the needle bar is attached to the end of the armature bar, so the needle is pushed down and into your skin. The instant the needle pushes down, the electric circuit is broken. The magnets turn off and the armature bar and the needle go back up. This happens so rapidly, it creates the infamous buzzing sound you hear in every tattoo shop.

The needle pierces your skin approximately 50 times a second. Depending on the machine, the tattoo design, and the tattooist, that number varies. Some tattooists like to run the machine faster while others prefer a slow and steady technique.

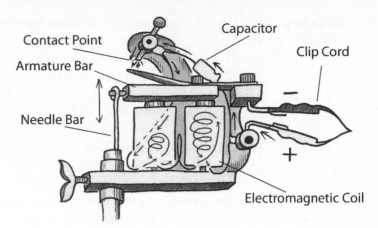

Contact Point

Armature Bar

Needle Bar

Capacitor

Clip Cord

Electromagnetic Coil

Machine operation.

You Needn't Be Afraid of Needles

You don't need to be afraid of this needle. It's completely different from the needles your doctor tortured you with when you were a small child. Hypodermic needles are really just sharp tubes designed to either take stuff from you, or put something in you. Tattoo needles are only for putting something in you, but unlike the hypodermic needles that go deep into your veins and body tissue, tattoo needles only go into your skin. Tattoo needles do not go very far into your skin, which we learned in the previous chapter.

Needles are very important in the tattoo process. They are the actual device that puts the ink into the skin and causes that lovely feeling of tattooing. They must be sterile and can only be used once on one person. They must be discarded after each use and stored in a *sharps container* until properly disposed of by a special waste disposal company. Luckily, needles don't cost very much at all, so it's no sweat just tossing them away.

def•i•ni•tion

A **sharps container** is a box, usually made of red or translucent white plastic, where used medical waste that can puncture or cut the skin, such as a needle, is disposed of.

def•i•ni•tion

Pins are the smaller, individual needles that are soldered together to make a tattoo needle.

Tattoo needles are made up of smaller *pins*, which are soldered together in a grouping. The grouping is then soldered to a needle bar, which gives the needle that long shape. This can be a time-consuming process and is why some old-timers used to use the same needle all day and only make a new one when that needle was too dull to pierce the skin. Laws have been put in place to keep people from doing that. Of course, by today's standards with today's diseases, the idea of reusing a needle is disgusting. Tattoo artists can now simply buy new needles from the many supply companies available. It is easy and cheap to purchase ready-to-use tattoo needles of all different sizes.

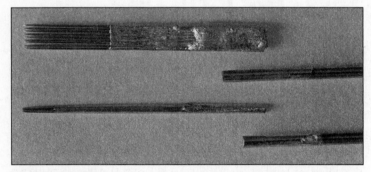

Needle grouping.

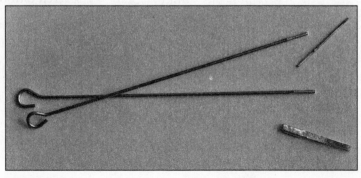

Needle bar.

Some artists still choose to make their own needles, which enables them to customize each needle the way they prefer it. There is a whole line of products tattooists can buy that allow the making of needles to be much easier and faster.

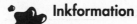

Inkformation

Needle-making is a skill that many younger tattooists don't bother to learn. The price of a premade, presterilized needle has gone down from $3 to less than 50 cents.

There are two basic kinds of needles: liners and shaders. There is one needle for making the outline of the tattoo, and one needle to fill in or shade the tattoo. Many artists, depending on the design, will use different sizes of lining needles to have varied thicknesses in the line weight of the tattoo. Some artists also like to have a small shading needle set up so they can get into the small areas, and a larger shading needle to fill in large open areas of the tattoo.

Liners

A liner needle is a group of pins that are soldered in a round formation. The needle grouping has to be a round shape or the lines of the tattoo will have an uncontrolled calligraphy to them. This may look very unprofessional and could ruin a customer's tattoo. The pins have to be in perfect alignment, or they will cause extra damage to the skin. This can cause the tattoo to heal weirdly and may possibly cause scarring. The last thing you want is a scarred tattoo.

As we have seen, there are so many different designs and styles in tattooing, as well as the different techniques to do them, that the liner needles must come in many sizes. Liner needles are categorized by the number of pins in the needle grouping. The number of pins in the needles runs from 1 to about 14 for liners. Some artists may use a larger needle than 14 for lining, but that is rare.

Shaders

Shading needles are flat and square-shaped like a flat paintbrush. They are wide in order to cover more space using fewer pins. The flat shape also helps to create smooth shading. A *magnum*

def•i•ni•tion

A **magnum shader** is a flat shading needle with the pins spread apart in order to make it easier to tattoo.

shader, or just "mag" as we say in the business, is the most used form of shader. Mags are good for filling in and shading because the pins are spread apart, so it's harder to chew the skin than if the pins were just flat across.

Shading needles come in many sizes, ranging from 4 to up to over 41. These large needles are the size of your thumbnail. They are generally only used for really large tattoos like a back piece.

Some shaders are round in shape like a liner and can be used to line as well. These are good for getting into little corners or to fill in up against a line. Some tattooists prefer round shaders for filling in tribal tattoos. It is up to the artist as to which shape of shader best fits the needs of the tattoo.

Tubes

The tube is the part that is held by the tattooist in his or her hands. It holds and guides the needle as well as gives the machine something to attach to. Tubes are the vessel for the ink from the ink cap to the skin. The tip of the tube, which is where the needle comes out, comes in different sizes in order to accommodate the different needles. After use, tubes are scrubbed and sterilized in order to be used again.

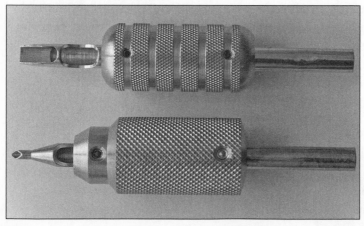

Tubes.

Some tattooists use disposable tubes. These are made entirely of plastic. They are good if a tattooist is on the road and doesn't have access to sterilization equipment, which we will go over later in the book. Plastic tubes can wear down quickly from the friction of the needle, which is problematic for use on long tattoo sessions.

A tube by itself is too thin and uncomfortable to hold. A device called a *grip* is used to give the tattooist a wider hold on the tube. Grips make it easier for a tattooist to control the direction of the needle. Grips come in different shapes and sizes. Some are made of stainless steel, while some are made to be lighter in weight by using aluminum or a hard plastic.

def•i•ni•tion

A **grip** is an attachment that serves as the "handle," enabling the tattooist to maneuver it more easily.

Those Nice Little Extras

Electric tattooing requires electricity and a way to control the electricity. As we know, a tattoo machine's speed is controlled by the amount of electricity running through it. A power supply is the device that conveys the electricity from the electrical outlet through a *clip cord* to the machine. It also enables the tattooist to control the speed of the machine with the simple turn of a knob.

def•i•ni•tion

A **clip cord** is the wire that attaches to the rear of the power supply by a plug or two clips, separated by a spring at the end of the cord.

Both of the tattooist's hands are in use during a tattooing session, so he or she uses a foot pedal to control the power. Like on a sewing machine, the tattooist uses the pedal to turn the machine on and off.

Some tattooists like to have the machine running constantly. They will rig the power supply to run the machine constantly without any foot pedal at all. This forces the tattooist to work faster.

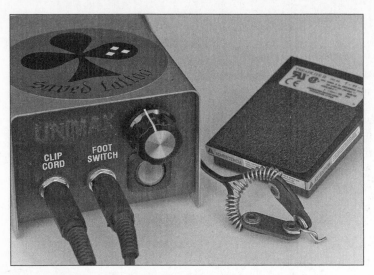

Power supply, foot pedal, and clip cord.

Sterilization

It is very important to have a clean and sterile environment for tattooing. Who wants to get tattooed in a dirty shop? Everything must be clean. The health department can shut a tattoo shop down for being dirty, and it's hard to tattoo if you don't have a place to do it.

The surface area in the tattoo station where your tattoo will be done must be sterile. Sometimes customers will not understand that their blood cannot get on anything, and will allow their bloody tattoo to touch a chair or an armrest. The area that is contaminated with the blood must be sterilized.

def•i•ni•tion

Matacide is a surface cleaner that kills germs and viruses such as *E. coli* or HIV.

To clean a surface properly, *Matacide* or a dilution of bleach is used. Matacide or the bleach dilution is sprayed on the contaminated surface, wiped down, and left for three to ten minutes to kill bacteria and viruses such as tuberculosis and Hepatitis C. The equipment a tattooist uses must also be clean and sterile. All of the needles and tubes must be sterile. There are two devices that are used to make sure your tattoo is clean and safe: the ultrasonic cleaner and the autoclave.

Ultrasonic Cleaner

In order to get all the particles out of a tube after use, a device called an ultrasonic cleaner is used. An ultrasonic cleaner is basically a small tub of water that vibrates all the particles out of the tube. Ultrasonic cleaners are also used to clean the dirt off of jewelry or the paint out of an airbrush. For tubes, a little hand scrubbing with a small brush is usually necessary to loosen up all of the particles. Then the tube is put back in the ultrasonic cleaner to get the rest of the microscopic particles out of the equipment. This ensures clean and safe equipment for every tattoo.

Autoclave

The ultimate machine in sterilization is the autoclave. A properly run autoclave will destroy every form of bacteria and virus with very, very few exceptions that we don't need to worry about. They are used in hospitals for sterilizing reusable equipment. Every tattoo shop should have an autoclave on the premises.

An autoclave works by heating water in a closed unit until it turns to steam. The steam then builds up pressure and heat in the contained unit, pushing all of the air out. The steam is heated to 121 degrees Celsius. Bacteria and viruses are then cooked to death as well as suffocated by the lack of oxygen. This lovely device allows tattooists to make sure their needles are sterile. Tubes will also be completely clean and ready to use without the risk of infection.

Ink

Ink is the actual component of the tattoo. Without ink, you would have to settle for branding and scarification. That just doesn't look as cool and it takes much longer to heal. One of the many trade secrets in tattooing is the ink. Where to buy the best ink, which will be the brightest, and which will last the longest are some of the great secrets. Today, with so many tattoo supply companies, it is easy to find colors and it is up to the tattooist to try to find the best.

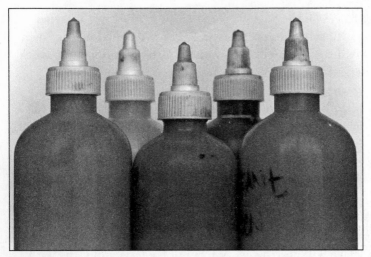

Inks.

Black

Black is the most common ink color used in a tattoo. It is usually used for the entire outline and for the dark shading. Many people choose to have their entire tattoo done in all black, such as with a tribal tattoo. Black will last the longest in the skin as it doesn't fade as fast as color can. Black makes the other colors stand out and look brighter.

The black ink used in tattoos is a carbon-based black. Carbon-based blacks are nontoxic so they're completely safe to use. Usually, some form of Indian ink is used for tattooing. All artists have their own formula for which black they use, so you may see a difference from one artist to the other.

Color

As with the black ink, tattooists have their own formula for colors. Most tattooists will purchase their inks from a supply company, which is quick and easy. There are many different colors available for tattooing. The variety of colors gives tattooists more freedom in coloring the tattoo.

Some tattooists will mix their own colors from nontoxic pigment powders. These pigments are mixed with water and alcohol until the artist gets the desired consistency.

Many artists prefer this method, so they know exactly what is going into the ink they are using.

Gray

Many people like to have only black and gray tattoos. Color is just not what they are looking for. Perhaps they are afraid the tattoo will be too bold and bright with color. Backgrounds for tattoos are usually done with a gray because gray isn't a strong color, therefore it will recede and let the other colors around it stand out. I have seen this with some Japanese tattoos where the backgrounds are done in black and gray.

Gray is an easy color to make. It is like an ink painting or an under-painting. Gray is just black watered down to a certain percentage for varying tones. Some tattooists will add some alcohol for antiseptic reasons. Another way to make a more opaque gray is simply to add a little black to white ink. This makes that battleship-gray tone, which can be slower to tattoo because it is thick but is brighter in the skin than just a gray wash.

The Least You Need to Know

- Modern tattoo machines are electric and vibrate tiny needles that introduce ink into the skin.
- There are basically two types of needles: one type for lining the tattoo and one type for shading the tattoo.

♦ Professional tattoo shops take great care to sterilize all equipment.

♦ Each tattoo artist has a unique way of working and mixing ink.

Chapter 6

Getting Serious

In This Chapter

- ◆ Forms and ID requirements
- ◆ Health concerns
- ◆ How much these things cost
- ◆ Appointments and consultations

Every industry has developed a certain way to do things, which makes the industry more efficient. It makes the life of everyone involved that much more convenient. The tattoo industry is no exception. A standard has grown that is fairly universal, give or take a little. In this chapter, we will go over some of the official procedures needed to get a tattoo as well as what some of the standards are today.

The Release Form

As you probably know, a tattoo is a permanent change to your body. There is no going back once the tattoo is done. Your skin is broken during the process, which makes it possible, although unlikely, for you to get an infection. It is because of these facts that some legal precaution must take place to protect the tattooist and the tattoo shop from lawsuits. Nobody likes being involved in a lawsuit unless you're talking about a lawyer.

A *release form* is the form you will need to fill out before your tattoo is started. It is necessary to fill out because it protects the shop legally. You are essentially legally giving the shop permission to tattoo you. This way there won't be any doubts if any problems, such as infection, were to occur later.

Release forms are really basic. They usually ask for your name, address, phone number, and e-mail. Then they ask if you have any allergies or a serious illness. You are informing the shop and the tattooist if you have anything that will complicate your tattoo process or if it's better that you didn't get tattooed. Release forms are also a good way for shops to keep track of customers just in case they need a better photo of the tattoo or just want to see how it healed.

Age and ID Requirements

It is important that you bring your ID when getting tattooed. In most states, the age requirement is 18. Some states, such as New Jersey, will allow a minor to get a tattoo as long as a legal guardian is there to sign. The legal guardian must have proof of guardianship and a photo ID.

> **Tattoo Taboo**
>
> Fake IDs will most likely be rejected. Most tattooists can tell what a fake ID looks like.

Most people use their driver's licenses for ID. For those nondrivers, a passport will do. You really just need some legal document with your birth date on it and preferably a photo.

Health Issues

There are certain situations in which you should not get a tattoo. As we have seen, the release form is designed to elicit information pertaining to that from you. In order to keep you from causing damage to yourself, tattooists will know the different scenarios that make tattooing dangerous to clients. It is hard to keep clients if they get sick or have bad reactions to a tattoo.

Sometimes you are just having health complications, which can happen to everyone. If this is the case, you may have to wait a little longer in life to get a tattoo. Some complications may never permit you to get a tattoo. It is always important to ask your doctor if you are physically able to get a tattoo. Let's look at the situations you should be aware of that may postpone your tattoo experience.

Pregnancy

While there is no evidence of direct danger that tattoos will affect your pregnancy or unborn child, most women are advised to delay their tattoo until after the birth. In fact, most tattooists will refuse to work on a pregnant woman.

Flash Tip

Henna, or mehndi, is a skin and hair dye that is used to decorate the skin for celebrations. It lasts anywhere from a week to a month, depending on the quality. It is used traditionally across the Middle East from North Africa to India. If you want to decorate your skin while you are pregnant, henna is the way to go.

Diabetes

If you have diabetes, it can be okay for you to get a tattoo. You should, of course, consult your doctor to be sure getting a tattoo is a good idea for you. But if you find that everyday pains like bumps and bruises are difficult to handle due to your diabetes, then you are better off not getting a tattoo. The risk of infection is much greater for people with diabetes.

Skin Complications

There are some skin complications that could keep you from getting a tattoo. Eczema, an inflammation of the skin such as a rash, should not be tattooed. It would be impossible to tattoo over the inflamed skin. Any really dry, crusty skin will be far too easy to damage while tattooing. Skin that is blistering, such as from poison ivy, will also not be able to be tattooed or even tattooed near. If you have a chronic form of eczema, you should consult your doctor before getting a tattoo.

People who suffer from psoriasis should not get tattooed. Psoriasis is a condition that affects the skin and joints. Patches of a person's skin appear red and scaly due to an overproduction of skin in those areas. Psoriasis can be very uncomfortable and the person suffering from it must be consistent with a healthy diet. Even alcohol can induce a breakout. The condition is not contagious but can spread on an individual if that person's skin is damaged. If an individual with psoriasis gets a tattoo, there is a possibility that tattooed area will form a plaque of psoriasis. This will consequently ruin the tattoo and will be very uncomfortable for the individual. It is not a good idea to get a tattoo while suffering with this condition, but definitely ask a doctor if you have both psoriasis and the determination to get a tattoo.

If you suffer from acne, you may want to wait until the acne has cleared up or you can find a place on your body that is pimple-free. Pimples, if tattooed over, can leave *holidays* in the tattoo when it heals. Then you will have to get a touch-up or just live with a tattoo with some imperfections. It's probably best to avoid an area with pimples and just get tattooed on the leg.

def•i•ni•tion

A **holiday** is a spot in a tattoo where the ink has fallen out during the healing process.

Moles

Moles occur due to a concentration of melanocyte skin cells, the melanin-producing skin cells we learned about in Chapter 4 This explains the dark color of moles.

A mole is best left alone or at least not tattooed over. Moles have a tendency to bleed profusely if they are cut or poked with a needle. It's not certain that tattooing over a mole will cause the mole to become cancerous, but moles are known to form melanoma, which is a dangerous form of cancerous melanocyte cells. It is the sun's UV rays that will cause the mutation of melanocytes to become malignant by altering the cells' DNA. When the cells divide in two, each new cell carries the malignant mutation. Moles can be an indicator of cancer through a color or size change.

Moles can often get in the way when designing a tattoo. It's best not to tattoo them because, if there is a mole in the way, there will be a hole in the tattoo. Many people like to have their moles incorporated into a design and disguised by a tattoo. When choosing the area of your body you want tattooed, try to find a place clear of moles and other skin complications.

Serious Health Risks

There are some diseases that a tattooist must be very careful of. These diseases live in blood and other bodily fluids. They can be transferred from person to person through *cross contamination*. Cross contamination is when viruses or bacteria are transferred from one surface to another. Without the proper steps, such as the use of matacide as we have seen in Chapter 5, diseases could be spread through a tattoo. The best way to stop cross contamination is to simply not touch anything that isn't protected by a disposable cover while tattooing.

def•i•ni•tion

Cross contamination is when contamination like the bloody ink wiped off a tattoo, is spread to another surface or substance through physical contact such as the touch of a bloody glove.

Anyone who has contracted HIV, Human Immunodeficiency Virus, should talk to a doctor before getting a tattoo. HIV is a virus that attacks the helper T cells in your blood. Helper T cells are the police of your immune system and usually take care of infections. Without these cells, your body becomes susceptible to infection. The infected state is called Acquired Immunodeficiency Syndrome or AIDS. It will be another disease that does the dirty work, HIV just opens the door.

Most tattooists won't tattoo anyone with the disease. The social stigma from HIV is very predominant in the tattoo industry because the industry has been a scapegoat for the spread of diseases in the past. HIV is actually very easy to kill once it is outside the body. It will die when it hits the air, but it can be lodged in small crevices in a drop of blood. Most cleansers will kill the HIV virus and matacide will take it down easily.

The disease that tattooists worry about the most is Hepatitis C. Hepatitis is a term used to describe an inflammation of the cells in your liver. It can be brought on by drug and alcohol abuse, the digestion of a poisonous mushroom, cancer, and many other situations. The symptoms of Hepatitis are flu-like. Also a person will get jaundice, the yellowing of your skin and eyes from bilirubin, a byproduct of the death of red blood cells, which also causes the yellowing of a bruise.

Most people in America have had their immunization shots for Hepatitis A and B. If you haven't gotten them, you should get them as soon as you can. Hepatitis C, however, has no preemptive cure and can stay in the body unnoticed (and able to be spread) for years and possibly decades. It is spread through contact with blood or through unprotected sex. It is estimated that four times the amount of people are infected with Hepatitis C than are infected with HIV. Depending on the state, 20 to 60 percent of prisoners in the penal system are infected with Hepatitis C.

Hepatitis C can survive on a counter top for over 11 days and still infect someone if it gets in his or her blood. This is why it is so utterly important that you go to a clean and reputable tattoo shop. If you have Hepatitis C, you will want to ask your doctor about getting your tattoo. Like HIV, you may find it hard to locate a tattooist who is willing to tattoo you.

Scars

Scars can be a bit tricky to tattoo over. As we discussed in Chapter 4, scar tissue is different from regular skin. There are a few things you need to know about getting scar tissue tattooed.

First, a scar from some form of surgery must be fully healed in order for it to hold ink. A scar that is tattooed over too soon can get worse and be more sensitive. Usually a year of healing will do for really deep scars. If you feel the scar is still too sensitive, wait until it seems ready or ask your doctor.

Second, the tattoo will only go over the scar; the texture of the scar will always be there. There are many different treatments for reducing the appearance of scars, such as laser surgery or dermabrasion.

Third, scar tissue can be thick, and it may take a couple of different sessions with the artist to get the ink in. Everyone heals differently when it comes to tattoos, so it's hard to say if the tattoo will stick the first time.

Flash Tip

Tattoos over stretch marks work just fine with a few precautions. The skin in a stretch mark is thin and easy to overwork if the tattooist isn't careful. Stretch marks can balloon up while they are being tattooed, but return to normal after a short time. The skin of the stretch mark will also bleed a little more than usual right after being tattooed.

Price Range

Different parts of the world will charge different amounts for tattoos. Some places are cheaper than others. Usually countries with weaker economies have much cheaper tattoos. The same goes with cities and towns. Higher rent for a shop will lead to higher cost for tattoos. Also a tattooist who has more experience and is faster will most likely be more expensive than a beginner.

There are a few ways tattooists figure out how much a tattoo is going to cost. It all depends on what the design is, how big it is, and where on the body you want the tattoo. In some shops, the designs may already have prices on them so you can just see for yourself. The three basic ways a tattooist creates the price is by the piece, by the hour, or by the shop minimum.

Per Piece

One way to price a tattoo is to charge one flat price for it. This is usually used for small to mid-sized pieces because the tattooist already knows how long it will take and how much effort the design needs. Placement is key because some spots on the body, such as the stomach, take longer to tattoo. The longer the tattoo takes, the more it will cost.

Tattoo Taboo _____

If you feel you have been given an exaggerated price, it's best to quietly go to another shop and ask them about the same kind of design. You may find that you just thought the tattoo would be less expensive than it is. You might prefer to go back to the first shop.

For larger tattoos, some tattooists will charge per session. That is a flat rate for a certain period of time. It is easy to work this way if you don't like being run by a clock. Instead the tattooist goes by how much tattooing is to be completed as opposed to how much time was spent.

Flash design that would have a flat price and be done in one session. Design by John Reardon.

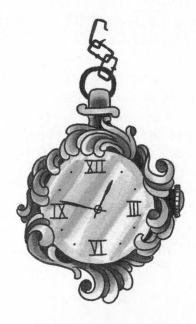

Per Hour

Many shops prefer to charge by the hour. This way the clock tells you how much to pay, and it is easier to know how much you will be charged. For ongoing tattoos, which take months to complete, the client can reserve a certain amount of hours per session. Usually it's at least two hours, but not more than four, depending on the tattooist and the client.

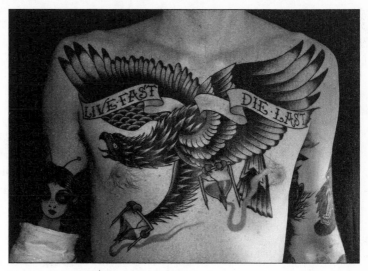

Large per-session tattoo done by Eli Quinters,
www.tattoosfortheunloved.com.

Shop rates in the United States run somewhere from $100 to $200 an hour. The average hourly rate is $150. The more popular shops are $180 to $200 per hour. It all depends on who is tattooing you. Remember that good tattoos aren't cheap.

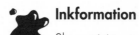

Inkformation

Shop minimums range from $40 to $100 for small tattoos on easy-to-tattoo places on the body, and the minimum cost covers black ink only.

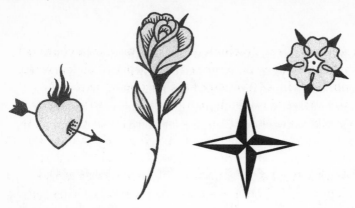

Minimum-priced tattoo designs.

Getting Started

When getting a tattoo, many shops will have you make an appointment. If you go into a busy street shop and they are too busy to tattoo you at that time, they may have you make an appointment for later in the day. Sometimes you may need to wait a week or two. If you are interested in getting a custom tattoo, in which the artist must draw your design, they will take a deposit and set you up with a consultation so the tattooist can create your drawing. Let's take a look at these aspects of the tattoo process.

Consultations

If you want to get a custom-drawn tattoo, you will first want to set up a consultation with your tattooist. This is a good time to get to talk with your tattooist about the design you want to get. You can explain why you are getting this design and what influenced you to get it. If you have any images showing different versions of your design, now is the time to give them to the tattooist. It's kind of fun and exciting, and you can drink a coffee while you have an open discussion.

Your tattooist will use this time to get to know you a little better so he can brainstorm the right vision and style for you. From his interaction with you, he can tell how serious you are (or aren't) about the tattoo. He can judge your level of commitment to following through with the full process of the tattoo.

Tracings

The tattooist may take a tracing of the area you want to have tat-tooed. Tracings are done on either tracing paper or plastic wrap. Some tattooists will take a photo of the area being tattooed to reference the curves of the body part. This is also so that they have the correct dimensions; this way they won't have to redraw the design if it is too big or too small. Tracings help out most when there are other tattoos to be tattooed around. If you are covering another tattoo, the tattooist will trace the old tattoo. Having a copy of the old tattoo shows the artist what is needed to cover it up.

Deposits

To hold an appointment or to have a drawing started, you will need to leave a deposit. This is to make sure you are coming back and the tattooist isn't sitting there without someone to tattoo. If you don't show up, the tattooist will at least keep the deposit and hopefully someone else will come in for her to tattoo.

The amount of the deposit differs from shop to shop. If a draw-ing isn't necessary because you are getting a design off the wall, some shops will only ask for a $20 deposit, and it will be deducted from the price of the tattoo when it is done. Many shops only ask for $50 while some tattooists will ask for at least $100 if there is a large drawing involved.

Many tattooists will deduct the deposit of a large tattoo from the very last session. This is to keep you coming back, as many people move away or are just too busy with their lives to fin-ish their commitment. Also, if a client doesn't show up for one of his or her appointments, the client can lose the deposit and will have to put down another one to make more appointments.

Flash Tip

Most tattoo shops will understand if a medical or family emergency keeps you from coming to your appointment. Just call them and let them know as soon as you are able to and you won't lose your deposit.

It's rare, but some tattooists use the deposit as a drawing fee. This makes sense if the drawing is going to take many hours of drawing and studying to complete. People seem to appreciate things more when they pay for them.

Drawings

In the consultation, you described your ideas as fully as you can to the tattooist. The tattooist should have a very good understanding of what you are looking for. It should be easy enough for him to start putting your drawing together.

Many tattooists don't charge for the drawing of a tattoo. They take on the challenge of drawing for you because they believe you are going to get the tattoo. Not many people realize that a tattooist can spend up to six hours or more drawing one design. This is out of his own personal private time. If the tattooist is drawing a subject matter he hasn't drawn before, it can take him much longer to draw. Also, drawing a cover-up so an old tattoo is "gone" takes an immense amount of work and concentration. This is where tattooing becomes more of an art than a craft, and an art background really makes the difference.

When you come in to see the drawing, the tattooist, if she is there, will study your reaction to know if something needs to be changed. Many tattooists will redraw the design for you if they need to, but only to a certain point. If it's a large drawing, it's not too kosher to add or change the ideas of the drawing after it has been completed. Most artists don't mind a little change, but to redo the whole thing because of a last-second change of mind defeats the whole purpose of the consultation.

Many tattooists will not let you leave the shop with the design or a copy of the design. Many clients ask to do this and often get cross when they are told they cannot. If the design goes out the door, the person with the design can then bring it somewhere else to get it tattooed. You may think that is preposterous but it happens all the time. They will get it tattooed cheaper in another shop by someone with less talent.

Scheduling

When getting a tattoo, you don't want to feel rushed or feel like you have to tell the artist to hurry up because you have to be somewhere. It's a much nicer experience to be able to sit and not worry about the time. It's a good idea to always book the correct amount of time for your tattoo. Set your day up so you have enough time. Remember, the tattoo is permanent so take your time.

Many tattooists have a habit of running a little behind on time. Sometimes they are behind by a few hours and you may find yourself waiting for your appointment. It's a good idea to not make any other appointments for yourself on your day to get tattooed. In addition, getting tattooed can wear you down and make you a little impatient. It's best to plan your day to be stress free so you can be relaxed for your tattoo.

> **Inkformation**
>
> The time a tattoo will take is very unpredictable. Like at a doctor's office, be prepared to wait your turn.

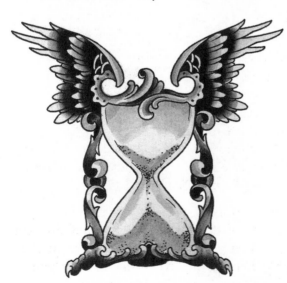

Time can be unpredictable in a tattoo shop so plan for more than enough. Flash by John Reardon.

The Least You Need to Know

◆ You will need to fill out a release form every time you get tattooed.

◆ In most states and countries, you must be at least 18 years of age to get a tattoo and have a picture ID.

◆ There are serious health conditions that may prevent a person from getting tattooed.

◆ The pricing of a tattoo will vary from tattooist to tattooist, but the average hourly rate is $150.

◆ For custom tattoos, you may need a consultation so you and your tattooist can go over your idea.

◆ Planning and scheduling should be as flexible as possible.

Part 2

Beginning the Tattoo Process

You most likely were ready to get a tattoo the moment you opened this book, but now you are better informed and better prepared. Let's get your tattoo process started.

This part covers the actual process of getting a tattoo. It's a guide to help you choose the correct design so you don't have any regrets. And you'll learn how to find the right tattooist who will ensure you a good experience and a great tattoo.

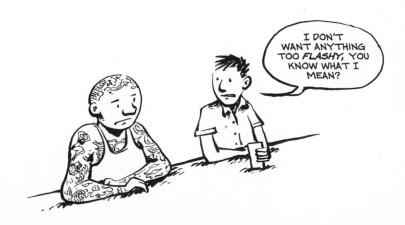

Chapter 7

What Works and What Doesn't

In This Chapter

- How the medium of skin determines design
- Concepts to avoid when getting a tattoo
- What a tattoo needs
- Design concepts of good tattoos

In choosing a tattoo design, the medium of the skin must play a factor. Good tattooists will understand how a tattoo grows and ages with the individual. They will know how to design a tattoo so it will look good after it has healed, as well as 30 years from the initial tattooing. It may seem hard to imagine yourself aging, but time is an unchangeable factor of life and so is the aging of your tattoo.

In this chapter, we will go over the different standards that tattoo designs must have in order to age well. You will learn what can and can't be tattooed and a few tips as to the concepts of what makes for good tattoo designs. When you enter the tattoo shop to talk to the tattooist, you will be prepared to talk about tattoo designs.

Skin Is Not Paper

Inking in skin is very different from inking on paper. As we saw in Chapter 4, tattooing is poking holes in the skin while forcing ink into those holes to leave a visible mark. Hence, the act of tattooing involves depth, whereas a tattoo on paper is just drawn on the surface.

When drawing on paper you can use a lightweight pencil, while a tattoo machine can be quite heavy and will also have the clip cord dragging off the back of it. It also vibrates while in use. These are a few things you need to understand in order see why certain things just aren't possible to do in the tattoo medium that could easily be done on paper.

Skin Moves When You Move

Skin is one large organ. As we saw in Chapter 4, it is the largest organ in the body. It is a cover that stretches, bends, squishes, and twists with your every movement. Your tattoo will also squish and bend when you do.

Take a look at the first knuckle on your right index finger. Point your finger straight and you will see your skin bunch up and appear wrinkly. Now bend your finger. You will see the skin stretch out and become relatively flat. While your finger is bent, take a non-toxic marker and draw a line over the top of that knuckle so it runs down toward your fingernail. Now straighten your finger. You will see that the line from the marker is now much shorter.

The stretch and squish will happen at different rates of movement all over your body. Your tattoo will look normal while your body is in one position, then it will stretch and warp when in another position. For this reason, and as we will see in Chapter 12, your tattoo stencil will most likely be put on your body while you are standing.

Skin Ages

Tattoos are permanent, and as we have seen, the tattoo will become a part of you. As you grow older and your body and skin change, your tattoo will change and grow with you. If you have a parent, grandparent, or even a friend with an older tattoo, you will be able to see what a tattoo grows or ages into. You can see how, as we saw in Chapter 4, the ink has receded in the skin and spread out, appearing faded and blurry.

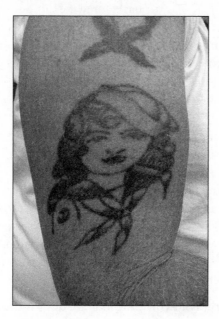

Notice how the lines have spread and faded, making the image look blurry. This tattoo on my father was done in 1960.

Aging of the skin and the result that has on the tattoo are partly the reasons why tattoo designs have to have a certain criteria in order to look good. An older tattoo will appear lighter and much softer. Lines that are too close together may blur into one line. Small spaces of untattooed skin that is surrounded by tattooed skin will begin to close in and disappear. The entire tattoo will slowly and subtly expand like a sponge in water. If there are any sharp points in the tattoo design, they will lose their sharp appearance. The color will slowly lighten up. The entire tattoo will appear more blurry and out of focus.

> **Flash Tip** _____
>
> Moisturizing your tattoo on a regular basis will help to keep your tattoo from prematurely aging. Keeping your skin moisturized will keep it healthy, which means your tattoo will stay in good condition.

It takes about a decade before any real signs of aging begin to appear in your tattoo, depending on how you take care of it and if you keep it out of the sun. Some people decide to have old tattoos done over. Some people with lots of coverage will start on a second layer when the older tattoos have lightened up enough to have a new tattoo put over them. Usually the first layer will consist of unwanted tattoos. Most often people are happy with the aged tattoos, as they are a reminder of younger days, marking a period of that person's life.

All Skin Is Different

Skin is as varied as individual personalities. Some skin is thick and stretchy, and some is tight and paper-thin. As you know, the color of skin varies also. From Chapter 4, you will remember that the amount of melanin produced by your skin determines the color. The melanin is produced above where the tattoo ink becomes trapped, so it will partially block the reflection of light from the tattoo. For this reason, color is not suggested for really dark-skinned people. Red will usually show the best on dark skin, but it won't be very bright.

If you are really dark, you will want to get a design that is very high in contrast with a good balance between deep black shading and untattooed skin. Skin tone is brighter than tattooed skin, so untattooed skin will help in creating a tattoo with a higher contrast. You will want to get a thick outline, as thin outlines will be hard to see or go unnoticed. Large, simple designs are best, as they will be easier to see. For lettering, it's a good idea to get it large and use a thick outline and a little shading. Solid lettering on really dark skin may just look like black blobs.

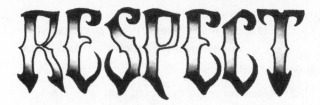

A good example of lettering that will work well on dark skin.

Medium-dark skin won't show color very well, either. The colors that will work best are blues and reds. If you remember from art class, blue and red are primary colors, which can't be made from combining other colors. This makes them stronger and brighter. Purple and green will work, but the colors can't be dark or they will look black. Usually adding a little white to the colors will brighten them up in the darker skin. On some dark-skinned people, yellows and oranges have worked, but it is rare. The odds are against these lighter colors working, but it's your decision if you want to try. Most of the time yellow and orange can hardly be seen once the tattoo heals, but there are always exceptions.

For olive-toned or really tanned skin, most colors will work fine. It is better to stay away from large fields of yellow and orange, as tanned skin is already orange in hue. It's like orange marker on orange paper. It won't stand out and may appear faded or invisible. With olive or tanned skin, it is better to have a tattoo based on a cool color such as blue, green, or purple if you want your color to stand out.

Very light-skinned people will have very brightly colored tattoos. The less melanin in your skin, the more light can reflect off the ink in your skin. If you don't want the tattoo to be bright but you are pale as a ghost, then you can have the tattooist use more white in the ink color. This will make the color more pastel, but it will also lower the color's intensity.

The skin on the different parts of your body will differ also. For example, the skin on your ribs is very stretchy and quite rubbery. It is difficult to tattoo due to its consistency. Also, the area is very sensitive, which can cause you to move around while being tattooed. It is not a good idea to get a tattoo with a lot of delicate lines in it on your ribs. It can be done, but it is very difficult on both the tattooist and the client.

The skin on the back of your neck is very thick as it covers your spinal cord. It is another place that is more difficult to tattoo. Much of the skin on the torso or around the elbows can take more time to tattoo as well.

Skin on the lower leg is often very taut and easy to tattoo. If you want a technical design with lots of lines and sharp corners, that is the place to do it. Forearms and the outside of the upper arm are also good spots to work on, as the skin is also easier to tattoo. The inner part of the upper arm is easy to tattoo but can be very sensitive. This is a good spot if you want your tattoo to be less noticeable, as the inside of your arm is often blocked from view.

Best if You Didn't ...

Not all tattoo ideas are good tattoo ideas. Tattoos are done by hand, so they will not be as perfect as if a computer printer made them. Also, the customer may move or shake a bit, which can also detract from near-perfection. Some designs are more susceptible to mistakes, especially if the client has a hard time sitting still.

The size and shape of the design can dictate its final outcome as well as its ability to age with grace. Let's take a look at some things to avoid when choosing your tattoo design. You and your tattooist will be much happier with your tattoo if you follow these guidelines.

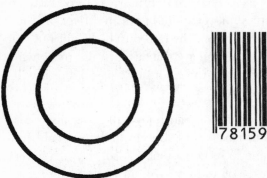

Here are some examples of ideas that do not work well as tattoos.

Perfect Circles and Parallel Lines

You will have a higher chance of success if you stay away from perfect circles. Try to draw one on paper. It isn't easy. Even Michelangelo used a circle tool such as a compass. There are no compasses for tattoo machines. Circles are done freehand with no physical guide other than a stencil. Any little bump in the line will stick out like a sore thumb. Also, due to the curves, angles, and movement of your body, the circle would really never look perfect.

It is possible to have a relatively perfect circle tattooed on you. However, you will need a very talented tattooist who will probably not want to tattoo it in the first place. You will also need to be absolutely still while the tattoo is being done. One little flinch and the whole thing can be ruined. You can have them done, but be prepared for it to look like it was done by hand. A little shading around the edge can help also. That way, any little twitchy part can be smoothed out. Many tattooists would prefer to not tattoo a circle and will try to talk you out of it or at least explain about possible imperfections.

Parallel lines are like circles: not easy to do and hard to fix if things go askew. Straight lines, like they were done with a ruler, are almost impossible to draw, let alone two of them right next to each other. Straight lines will also not look right on many parts of the body due to the body's curves and indents, as we shall see later in the chapter.

A popular idea for a tattoo is a barcode. This is a very good example of a bad design for a tattoo. First of all, the barcode won't ever work on an actual scanner. To tattoo a barcode, it has to be much larger than an actual barcode and have fewer lines. Considering that the entire design is nothing but straight parallel lines without any shading, the barcode is a very bad idea for a tattoo.

If the design is curved, it is possible to have an equidistant line around it. You are, however, opening yourself up to possible imperfections, which can be very noticeable. Shading placed in and around the lines to fix any imperfections would help out. Again, most tattooists will warn you about the dangers of parallel lines or just refuse to do the tattoo. It's best to choose a design that doesn't have these elements as the predominant aspect of the tattoo.

Geometrical Patterns

Geometrical patterns have some of the same problems as architectural designs do when it comes to tattooing. They may look really cool when they are printed out by a computer, and they may seem really simple, but try drawing them by hand. It becomes quite tedious and frustrating, and is almost impossible to do. Any repetition of any object is subject to slight imperfections.

Designs like checkerboards are very technical and are better if done in small doses. Checkerboard armbands are possible but not easy. As long as you understand that the tattoo will look like it was done by hand and not by a computer, then you are fine. But it may be a better idea to get designs that work best as tattoos, if you want your tattoo to look as good as it possibly can.

Too Small/Too Detailed

Lots of people just want a small tattoo to see if they can handle it. Small tattoos are generally quick and easy. You must understand that a small tattoo must be extremely simple. The line work of a tattoo has to be a certain thickness. And as we have seen, aging will blur the tattoo, so little details will be lost over time. Who wants a blob for a tattoo?

Many young women like getting fairies. Although many older women like getting their little fairies covered up with more mature tattoo ideas, young women still need their fairies. It seems to be an ongoing circle of life. Fairies are fine, but the major problem with fairies is that they have to be a certain size to get any detail in the face that will last over time. In order for the face of the fairy to look okay, it must be at least three quarters of an inch, and that is pushing it. It will still be very basic. The fingers, too, must be a certain size or else the fairy will have mittens.

Detail is nice in a tattoo but there is a limit. If the tattoo is over-detailed, it will be hard to read what is going on in the design. The detail will be lost. Little details may blur together over time, which will again leave you with an illegible blob. The larger the tattoo, the more detail you can fit in. Remember, detail is to accentuate the image as a whole, not to distract the eye from the main subject.

All Color

Tattoos that lack in black are a bad idea as far as lasting ability. As we explained earlier, color has a tendency to fade faster than black, and it can get blurry more quickly. Also, it is the contrast with the black ink that makes the color bright. Outlining in color is not a good idea, either. It is possible, but it will never be as bold as black, and it is also usually thicker and more difficult to line with. A little color outlining can be nice to enhance the tattoo design, but a tattoo will always look better and last longer with black as its base.

The White Tattoo

White tattoos are quite popular; however, this doesn't mean they are a good idea. If you really want an all-white tattoo, go for it, but there are a few things you should know first:

- ◆ White tattoos will often turn yellow, especially in the sun.
- ◆ Due to the friction of the needle against the tube, the white ink will turn slightly gray, leaving you with gray spots in your tattoo.
- ◆ To make a white tattoo look decent, they often have to be done twice.
- ◆ White tattoos are hardly noticeable in white skin, and will appear to look like scar tissue in dark skin.
- ◆ Many tattooists will just not do a white tattoo.

Fingers and Feet

Fingers are tricky spots to have tattooed. As explained in Chapter 2, getting a visible tattoo can cause problems for you in the work place or when you're out on the town. As accepted as tattooing is becoming, there are still those who are against it. Tattoos on the fingers are also more susceptible to infection, as you use your fingers to touch or hold various things throughout your day. Also, it is hard to keep them out of the sun's harmful UV rays. It is easy to knock off a scab by reaching into your pocket. A finger tattoo should only be done if you are ready to take care of it and if you are ready for the change it will cause in your life.

If you are going to get a finger tattooed, more power to you. The skin on a finger is different in that it will appear to age faster. Finger tattoos also have to be done twice due to your constant use of your fingers while they are healing. It is best to only get the tops of your fingers done, as the sides are hard to reach with the needle and don't hold ink well. The palm sides of your fingers don't hold ink well at all, as the skin is too thick. If you want a wedding-band tattoo, it's best to skip the palm side of your finger.

> **Flash Tip**
>
> After having your foot tattooed, it's best to have your feet out of your shoes as much as possible so the tattoo can heal. Try wearing flip-flops or something that won't rub against the tattoo.

The tops of your feet will hold a tattoo well as long as you take very good care of it. Toes, on the other hand, almost always have to be done a few times and the tattoo will still look old and blurry when it is done. Ink won't really stay in the bottom of your foot, and it would be excruciating to have it tattooed. It's better to stick to the top of your foot, above the toes, if you want the tattoo to look good.

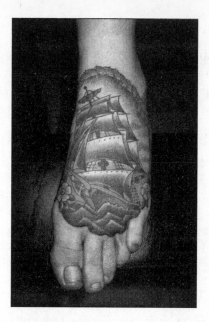

Foot tattoo by Amina Reardon, Tato Svend, Copenhagen, Denmark.

Better That You Do ...

As mentioned, tattoos can be quite painful, especially in certain areas, and they aren't cheap. This is why it is so important to do it right the first time. Tattooists who know what they are doing know that one of the most important and key factors to a good tattoo is black ink. It can't be stressed enough.

I mentioned in a previous section that color ink does not make for good outlines in a tattoo. Black outlines are very important to have. The black will stay in the skin and appear dark the longest. The outlines are the framework of the tattoo. They are the skeleton and will keep the design legible throughout the life of the tattoo. Tattoos look very faint without an outline. If it looks faint in the beginning, it will look even worse in a few years and you will have to pay to have it done again.

Many people have the false assumption that black shading will make the tattoo look too dark and heavy. Granted, too much black shading will do this, but having no black shading will do the opposite. The tattoo won't look as strong without the black. If you don't want a bold tattoo, that is one thing, but the tattoo will look amateurish if there isn't some kind of black base. You want to have the best-looking tattoo you can have, so stick with the black.

Better Design

Designing a tattoo is easy. Designing a good tattoo takes more effort and the guidance of experience. Both small and large tattoos need to have some basic guidelines for them to come out looking great. As we have seen previously, the designs need to be a certain size with a proportional amount of detail. This is to help with the aging of the tattoo. Let's look at a few concepts that will help you understand good tattoo design.

Fit It to the Body

When you look in the mirror, you will see that your body has lots of curves and plane changes. Your body has a certain shape. In designing tattoos, it's a good idea to keep this in mind and fit the design to these shapes. The tattoo could appear to clash with your natural shape and look awkward if it doesn't go with your flow.

Flash Tip

Just as a symmetrical design can look strange on an asymmetrical part of the body, an asymmetrical design can look strange on a symmetrical part of the body.

An example of this can be seen in symmetrical designs, that is, designs that are identical on both sides. Symmetrical designs will look awkward on a body part that is not symmetrical, such as an arm or leg. The static shape of the symmetry will conflict with the curved shape of the body part. Symmetrical designs work very well on symmetrical parts of the body, such as in the center of your back where the line of your spine is the centerline of the design. Also, the front of your torso will work well, such as on your chest.

A good shape that fits the body well is the *"s" curve*. When a design is based on an "s" curve, its flowing shape won't contrast to the curves of your body. The design will meld with the body's shape and movement. Many tattooists will fit the "s" curve directly to the curves of your muscles, such as where your deltoid muscle, or shoulder, curves into the beginning of

def•i•ni•tion

An **"s" curve** is a design concept in which the shape is based on the shape of an "s."

your biceps. If you must have a symmetrical design on an asymmetrical body part, you can have the artist put a little shading in an "s" curve shape behind the design. This will make the design fit much better and look more professional.

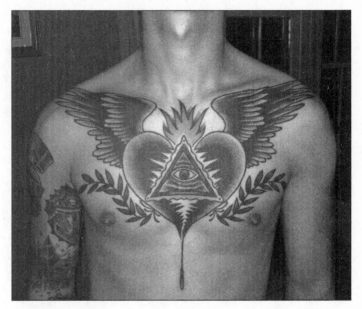

A symmetrical tattoo on a symmetrical part of the body. Tattoo by Chad Koeplinger, www.tattooparadisedc.com.

Facing the Right Direction

Some tattoo designs need to be facing a certain direction when placed on the body. Examples of this are designs that have a head or face, as well as designs that seem to be flowing or pointing in a certain direction. The general rule of thumb is to have the design facing forward. Your body is set up so that its forward direction is the belly side of your body, as opposed to a dog, whose belly is down but the head and shoulders face forward. So if you have a profile of a pinup or a woman's head, she would be looking forward toward the front of your body. This follows the flow of your body.

If the design is on either side of your chest, it is traditional to have the direction or gaze of the head face the center of your chest. The design should also face in a forward direction if it's on your ribs. On some occasions, you may specifically want the design to look behind you, or the design may call for the object to face a backward direction. That's fine, too, because as we have already seen, you are the one who needs to be pleased the most with the tattoo, and every design can call for something different.

The direction of the face in the design faces toward the front of the person's body. Tattoo by Steve Boltz.

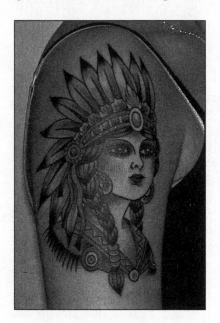

Planes of the Body

Just as your body has many curves and contours, there are also many flat spots or planes on your body. It is always best to place a tattoo on one of these planes so the entire tattoo can be seen at once. Of course, there are many designs that will wrap around the body, such as an armband, but for many tattoo designs, they will need to be on one plane to be able to tell what they are.

For example, a dragon's body can wrap around the arm, curving all over, but the head of the dragon is very important and needs to be seen clearly on one surface. It would be very awkward to only see half the head on one side of the arm, and then having to twist the arm to see the other half. The same goes with a portrait tattoo. The idea is to see the portrait in its entirety. A good tattooist will know the planes of the body and how to design your tattoo so that it will fit your body correctly.

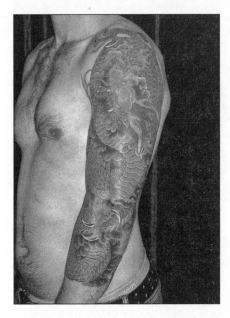

Notice how the body of the dragon wraps around the arm while the head of the dragon is clearly visible. Tattoo by Shinji (Horizakura).

There are many things that you need to keep in mind when looking for a tattoo or having one designed. Now you have a basic idea as to what will work and what to avoid. This will help you from choosing a design that may not age well and you may regret years later.

The Least You Need to Know

- ◆ Your tattoo will move, stretch, and age when you do.
- ◆ Certain colors such as red and light blue work best on darker skin.

- Tattoo designs that work best are designs that have more of an organic feel, as opposed to designs that are geometrical.

- For a tattoo to look the best it can, it must have black as a base and outline.

- Overall, the best design is the design that you love.

Chapter 8

Choosing Your Tattooist

In This Chapter

- ◆ Where to find a good tattooist
- ◆ Listening to the word on the street
- ◆ Will this fit in your schedule?
- ◆ Is this tattooist for you

Finding a good tattooist is very easy. There are so many good tattooists out there waiting to tattoo you. Unfortunately, there are also some bad ones. That is why it is important to take your time in finding the right person to tattoo you. You have your whole life to wear the tattoo. A few extra days waiting to find the person who will get the job done right isn't too much to ask. Perhaps you need to get the tattoo done quickly without a lot of mulling over the subject. Some people are like that, and that's fine, too. There is no need to worry as long as you take the right precautions when walking into a shop.

Many shops are designed for people to walk in and get a tattoo on the spot. Many of these places have amazing artists working there who will put a nice, clean tattoo on you. As long as you know what to look for, you won't have any mishaps.

Where to Look

It is time for you to start looking for the tattooist who is the best person for the job. There is a whole global community of them waiting for you to seek them out. Your tattooist is out there somewhere, and you will find that person. Now, where do you look?

If you have found the name of a tattooist or tattoo shop, you can then look it up on the Internet. Most shops have websites containing portfolios and photos of the shop. This way you can get a basic idea of the place without actually going there. (If you don't have access to the Internet, take the time to stop by and check out the shop.) If you can't get a referral from anyone, you can always look up local shops on the Internet. Google or Yahoo! are good places to start. MySpace also has many tattooists who have their portfolios posted in their photo sections. In addition, the artists who have contributed to this book are amazing tattooists, and this book is a good place to start looking.

Tattoo magazines will have pictures of tattoos with each artist's information. Many magazines will have full articles on the artists so you can learn about them before you meet them. This way you can see what the tattooists are into before you go out of your way to meet them.

Shop Reputation and Experience

One of the best ways to tell if a shop is good, bad, or ugly, is by its reputation. It takes years to build a good reputation, no matter what you do. A good reputation means happy clients, which means good tattoos. Because it takes years to build a good reputation it typically means a good reputation comes with experience. Experience is important because the tattooist will know what she's doing. She won't be experimenting or learning on you. She will know how to guide you through your tattoo experience and what to do in case of an emergency such as if you should pass out.

Many people find their tattooist through word of mouth. The best way to find a tattooist is to meet or know someone who has tattoos. It's hard *not* to find someone with at least one tattoo these days. Perhaps one of your co-workers or church buddies has been tattooed and can tell you about his or her experience.

Finding a tattooist through word of mouth also enables you to see the artist's work firsthand. It's good to see how a tattooist's work looks after it's healed. You can make your judgments without the pressure of being in a shop or in front of the artist.

If you see people in public with tattoos you think are nice, ask them where they got their tattoos. You will find many people get really excited to promote their tattooist. Many clients carry the cards of the shop where they got tattooed. Sometimes a referral may get them a discount on their next tattoo.

Inkformation

Being a tattooist is more than just doing some tattoos. Many tattooists choose their profession because they have been tattooed and because they want to become more tattooed. Not that the tattooist needs to have every inch of his body covered, but he should have a decent amount of tattoos. Having tattoos is a part of being a tattooist. A tattooist without tattoos is like a chef who doesn't know how his food tastes.

Availability

We all have our own lives and our own schedules of things to do, like doing the food shopping or going to Grandpa's birthday· party. It's a fact of life that sometimes you only get certain windows of time to get stuff done for yourself. When looking for a tattooist, you need to keep this in mind.

Appointments

It's not uncommon for a well-known tattooist to have a very busy schedule. Some tattooists are booked up for a year. Some are booked for six months, while others are just waiting for you to walk in. If you don't mind waiting, that's great, but it may be hard to plan your life a year in advance. There are too many things popping up to plan that far ahead.

It's good if you are sold on a particular artist and don't mind waiting for an appointment. Then you are all set. But if you don't have that kind of patience, it's best to look around to find someone who is available when you are. You want the experience to be a pleasurable one, so give yourself enough time to do things right.

Easy to Reach

Location is a big issue when you are looking for your tattooist. If you are getting a tattoo that takes more than one session, you may want to find a shop that is near where you live. If it takes you over an hour of travel to get to the shop, you may be tired by the time you get there. The more tired you are, the more the tattoo will hurt.

Traveling with a fresh tattoo can be uncomfortable also. Plus your tattoo will be bleeding on the way home. Being stuck on a bus or train during rush hour while you are recovering from a fresh tattoo is not fun.

Flash Tip

Try to ask around to see if the tattooist you're interested in is good about keeping appointments.

There are many tattooists who are worth traveling to get tattooed by. But because tattoos are not cheap to begin with, the additional costs of traveling a great distance and possibly needing to stay until the tattoo is finished can make the whole experience a huge financial commitment.

Personality

Because you are having someone change your body permanently, you may want that someone to be a person you like and trust. Having a pleasant tattooist can really make your tattoo experience a good one. Ask yourself the following questions:

◆ Do you feel comfortable? Feeling comfortable during a tattoo session is important. Feeling comfortable will keep you from jumping around during the tattooing process. What are your first impressions when you meet your tattooist? Some tattooists can look really burly on the outside but are friendly and understanding on the inside. You will have to spend some time with this individual, because you don't want to have a tattooist who gives you the heebie-geebies.

◆ Do you like the tattooist? It is always nice to hang out with people you get on with. They can make the time go by faster, which is important when you are getting a tattoo. When talking to a tattooist, ask yourself, "Is this person someone I could get along with outside the tattoo shop?" Not that you want to be best friends, but for the moment you are together, there won't be any hang-ups. You don't have to agree on everything, but it's nice to be around someone pleasant.

Style

For a tattooist to do the best job he can, he needs to want to do the tattoo you chose. Not all tattooists will tattoo anything. Some are quite specific about what they are willing to tattoo. Some have studied hard to tattoo a certain kind of style and don't want to be bothered with anything else. This is why it's important to do a little research before speaking to a tattooist. A tattooist's style is what sets his or her tattoos apart from everyone else's.

Flash Tip _____

It's a good idea to look at the tattooist's portfolio and see if the tattoos she has done look similar to what you want to have done so that the end results of your tattoo will look similar or better than what you had expected.

If the Idea Fits

Style can be very specific. Many themes and ideas can be transferred from one style to another. A good example of that can be seen in classic art. How many different artists for the last 2,000 years have painted the Madonna and Child? From Duccio to Raphael, the image has changed with each passing style and trend. It wouldn't fit so well or at least have the same meaning if someone like H. R. Giger painted the Madonna and Child. There is no way that painting would make it inside a church and no way any devout Catholic wouldn't be offended by the image Giger would make.

> **Flash Tip** _____
>
> It's a good idea to look at the tattooist's portfolio and see if the tattoos she has done look similar to what you want to have done.

With this in mind, you must ask yourself, while you are looking through portfolios, "Does my idea fit this style of tattooing?" Someone who tattoos graffiti isn't necessarily going to want to draw a tribal sun. You will probably find a similar version of your idea in someone's portfolio, so just keep looking.

Is the Tattooist Into Your Idea?

It's easy to tell if a tattooist is into your idea. You can usually see it in the expression on his face. That's why it's important to meet with him beforehand and discuss your plans. Forcing someone to do something artistic that he doesn't want to do can result in a bad tattoo. If he's not into your plan, then you can do one of two things:

1. If you really like this tattooist for personal reasons as well as liking his portfolio, you can ask him what he would rather do. From there you can go back and forth until you both are satisfied with your future tattoo. You will probably end up with a tattoo you love more than your original idea.

2. If you are really into your idea for a tattoo and must have that idea, you can ask the tattooist if he has a friend who can tattoo or a co-worker who may be into the idea. This enables the tattooist not to have to do something he doesn't like, as well as hook up a buddy or respected tattooist.

Cleanliness

To avoid any possibility of infection, make sure the shop you go to and the artist you want to do your tattoo are clean. It is not easy to infect a tattoo, but it is possible if the shop is dirty. Look for dust balls or ink stains on the floor. If the floor hasn't been mopped in a while, chances are nothing else has been cleaned either. A clean toilet is a sign of a clean shop. Being clean is another sign of a professional and a good sign of a competent tattooist.

You already know about the sterilization equipment and Matacide from Chapter 5. Make sure there is some form of Matacide or bleach cleaner kicking around the shop. That's a good sign that the shop is kept sterile. You should be able to smell the bleach or chemical cleaner in the air. They are unmistakable smells and point to a clean shop. Look for boxes of surgical gloves as well. These are also a sign of attention to cleanliness and detail.

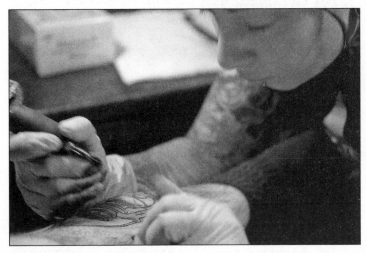

Tattooist working with gloves.

Check out the tattoo area while you are looking around the shop. If you see the garbage cans are overly full and appear to have been sitting around for a while, you may want to look somewhere else. The trash in the garbage will be contaminated with blood and dirty ink.

Single-Use Needles

Most tattooists use a needle only once and then dispose of it after the tattoo. It is very rare that someone will reuse a needle as it is highly frowned upon in the tattoo industry. Still, to be sure, ask the tattooist if the needles are single use. If he says no, run for the hills.

Tattoo Taboo

It is very, very rare that a tattooist will use a used needle, but it still may happen. Ask to see the needle taken out of the autoclave package while the tattooist is setting up.

To be 100 percent sure, you can ask the tattooist if you can watch him take the needle out of the package. Be sure to do that before the tattooist starts to set up for you so you can watch.

If you remember from Chapter 5, tattoo needles are relatively inexpensive these days and are very easy to buy for the educated professional. Reusing needles is very rare and would be more of a pain for the tattooists than to just buy new ones.

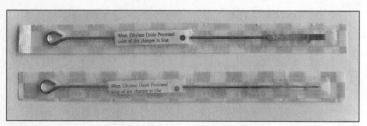

An example of new sterilized needles in sealed packages.

The Least You Need to Know

- ◆ Recommendations and seeing tattooists' work first hand is the best way to find your artist.

- ◆ Be sure to meet with the tattooist, look at his or her portfolio, and discuss your plans first.

- ◆ Having a good professional rapport with the tattooist will make your tattoo experience a little easier.

- ◆ Cleanliness with tattooists is a sign of professionalism and makes for a better tattoo.

9

Quality Control

In This Chapter

- ◆ What to look for in a portfolio
- ◆ How to determine good line work
- ◆ What a solid tattoo looks like
- ◆ How to see if a tattoo is overworked

If you are going to get a tattoo, you might as well get it done right. From the previous chapters, we learned how to make sure you get a clean, safe tattoo as well as where to find an artist. Now let's see what makes a tattooist good. It makes sense to try to have the best when it comes to permanently changing your body. You have to live with the tattoo for a long time, so you'll want to make it a good one.

In this chapter, we will go over the different aspects of a tattooist's work. We will learn how to break down the technical ability of a tattooist through examining his tattoos to see if he is the right one to do your tattoo. After reading this chapter, you will be able to see if a tattooist is experienced or if he is going to leave you with a scar and a headache, instead of a tattoo.

Looking at Portfolios

A portfolio is the professional representation of the tattooist. It portrays the artist's ability to tattoo and is a sign of how committed she is to the profession. Through looking at the portfolio, you will be able to determine the artist's style. You can see the level of ability of the artist and determine whether or not your tattoo is a good idea for this particular person to execute.

However, some of the best artists do not care about portfolios. They are usually rather busy and don't have time to prepare one or keep an existing portfolio updated. The portfolios of these talented artists are walking around on the street, and you are lucky if you get to see one of these amazing pieces. For the beginner, always choose a tattooist with a portfolio. Once you are more familiar with the process or have an ongoing relationship with your tattooist, seeing a portfolio might not be necessary.

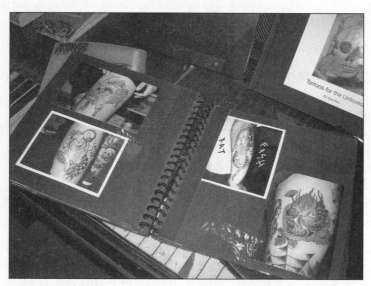

Sample portfolios.

Presentation

The first thing you will notice about the portfolio is its appearance. There are many different kinds of portfolio cases ranging from overpriced art store portfolios to family photo binders from the dollar store. Both work just fine and the really important part is the tattoos inside. Regardless, one can get a feeling of what to expect from the kind of portfolio. The large fancy ones are sometimes a sign that the tattooist is making up for something. Like when men have to drive large trucks or fancy sports cars. Don't let the ostentatious façade keep you from seeing what's on the inside. Having a fancy portfolio case can also be a sign that the tattooist cares for what they are doing. He puts in the extra effort.

Having a cheap or beat up and worn down portfolio can be a sign that the tattooist doesn't care. If he is not willing to put the effort into the portfolio, will he put the effort into the tattoo? Cheap portfolio cases, on the other hand, are often a response to customers destroying previous portfolio cases. Many people find it necessary to man-handle the portfolio while looking through it, whipping through the pages like the book was an ex-lover who left with the mailman. Often people will spill drinks on them and not clean them up. Many tattooists tattoo people all day and not one of those people bothered to look at the portfolio. It sounds ridiculous but these things happen all the time, so many tattooists will give up on the portfolio case after replacing it so many times.

A portfolio's appearance will vary from shop to shop and tattooist to tattooist. If it impresses you, then great, go for it. Just remember, the contents are the most important factor for the conclusions you need to make.

All Those Wall Designs

While looking through a portfolio, one of the ways to see if a tattooist will be able to tattoo a more specific design or come up with a custom design is to see if most of the designs in the portfolio are designs from the flash on the wall. It's expected that there will be a few. Some flash designs are really fun to tattoo and look really cool. It's fun for a tattooist to tattoo designs from other artists.

Many tattooists only tattoo flash designs and are amazing technical tattooists. If what you want is a design from the wall or a specific design that doesn't need to be customized, you are in good hands with these individuals. However, too many flash designs in a portfolio are a sign that the tattooist either won't draw a custom tattoo or just can't.

Draftsmanship

While looking through the portfolio, you will want to study the tattooist's ability to draw. If the designs look a little kooky, like the face on a portrait or a pinup looks like it got kicked by a mule or spawned by Sloth from the movie *The Goonies,* then you may want to move to the next portfolio. Even with an untrained eye, there is a certain level of poor draftsmanship everyone can see. You will be able to feel if a drawing is really unbalanced or the perspective is wrong.

> **Tattoo Taboo**
>
> The tattooist's ability to draw is important if you are looking for an original design or image. Ask to see sketches of other designs before you commit.

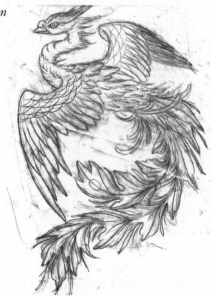

Drawing of a design by John Reardon.

Blurry Photos

Blurry photographs will make it impossible for you to see if the tattoo is any good or not. You will need to be able to see the tattoo clearly in order to see if you like it. If the portfolio is full of horrible photos, it may be a sign that the tattooist is trying to hide something, like the fact that she is not very accomplished at tattooing.

Many professional tattooists will invest in a good camera. Some studios have a small section in the shop set up as a photo studio with lights and a backdrop. With digital photography improving every year, many tattooists only need a small digital camera to take a decent photo. You don't need as much light with digital cameras as they are getting better at compensating for amateur photographers. Digital cameras also make it easier to put photos instantly on the Internet. A tattooist is not a professional photographer so don't expect perfect photos. The photos should at least be in focus so you can see the quality of the tattoo. Polaroids just won't cut it.

Originality, Not Quantity

It may happen that a tattooist who is not as serious may want to try to fool the customer by having an excessive amount of photos in his portfolio. He thinks that quantity will make up for a lack of quality. Usually with portfolios that consist of mostly flash pieces, there will be the same piece of flash tattooed at a different time on a different person. This is unnecessary and a sign that the tattooist didn't have anything better to display.

If you have ever been to or applied to some form of art school or design job, you will know that to determine the skill of an individual, you only need 15 to 20 pieces. Quantity will become overkill.

> **Inkformation**
>
> While you are looking through a portfolio, remember that it is the quality of the tattoos that is important, not the quantity of tattoos.

In tattooing, it is nice for people to see the different designs that can be tattooed and what they look like in the skin. Lots of clients will choose a tattoo from the portfolio. In this case, the portfolio is like a wall of flash and that works, too. There is no need to put the same design twice on the wall, so there is no need to put a design twice in the portfolio.

There are a few tattooists, like the famous Horiyoshi III of Yokohama, Japan, who will have huge portfolios full of numerous tattoos. He has been tattooing for decades and has completed numerous bodysuits and other large tattoos. The tattoos, due to their size, need to be photographed from many different angles to show all the different aspects. Portfolios like this are more like a museum of mastered tattooing and can take hours to look through to really appreciate the work. In this case, a portfolio becomes a tattooist's legacy.

When Tattoos Look Worse Than the Originals

While checking out a portfolio, you recognize a piece of flash that has been tattooed and can find the original in the flash. Go ahead and compare the two. If you are just starting to look at tattoos and portfolios and feel a little overwhelmed by the experience, comparing a tattoo with the original design can be a good way to get your ground.

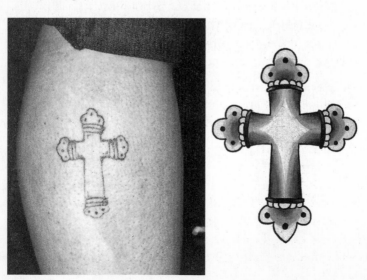

A bad tattoo and good flash.

You will be able to see if the tattooist can reproduce a design on the skin. You will be able to see if mistakes were made or if the shading is off. Keep in mind that some tattooists like to change the design a little while they are tattooing. It can make doing the tattoo more fun for the tattooist, as customers choose many of the same flash designs over and over again. The tattooist may have put a flash tattoo in his portfolio that he purposefully changed to show that a tattoo could be more custom.

Are You Impressed?

The purpose of looking through a portfolio is to find a tattooist who you want to do your tattoo. The portfolio of your tattooist should make you feel comfortable that you are going to get a high-quality tattoo from this person. You need to have confidence in the tattooist's ability to work. Trusting in your tattooist will help you relax before and during the tattoo. You will sit for the tattoo much better and the process will be easier on the both of you.

Line Work

The very base of every tattoo is the line work. It is the frame of the tattoo. It will guide the placement of the shading and the coloring. The line work will hold the tattoo together as it ages over the years. It will keep your tattoo legible after 30 years.

Good, clean line work is a sign of years of experience and of confidence with the needle. It takes some time for a tattooist to develop clean lines, usually at least five years of experience on average. With good training in the apprenticeship and the occasional "gift from God" of talent, it can take less time to perfect good line work. Really good tattoo machines help, too.

It is nearly impossible for the line of every tattoo a tattooist does to be utterly perfect. Every customer has a tendency to move now and again. Also, some people's skin is very difficult to tattoo. Certain parts of the body, like the ribs, are just really hard to tattoo. This is why tattooists try to discourage tattooing perfect circles or parallel lines. It's not that it isn't possible, it's just that the odds are against perfection even from the most experienced tattooist.

A tattoo outline by John Reardon.

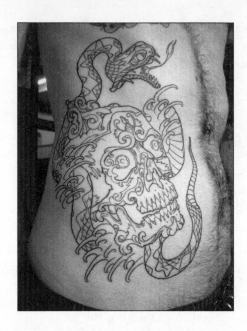

Some tattooists develop a style where the line work is done very quickly and the tattooist doesn't pay too much attention to the quality of the line. This is more relevant in large tattoos such as a back piece. The shading and the coloring will cover much of the lines so you won't really notice unless you get really close.

> **Flash Tip**
>
> If you do jump or move a bit during a tattoo and cause a squiggle in the line, don't worry too much. Ninety-nine percent of the time the imperfection in the line can be covered with the shading.

While looking at a tattoo, there are a few things to look out for. They are common mistakes that happen to every tattooist now and again. However, an overabundance of them is a sign of someone you don't want to get tattooed by. Let's take a look so you will know them when you see them.

The Shakes

The last thing you want is a shaky tattoo. Shaky line work will ruin your tattoo. Some imperfections in the line can look fine, as tattoos are done by hand, not a computer printer. But too many of them may make you quite unhappy, especially if they are in really important spots, like the nose of a pinup girl or the mast of a ship. When you look at a portfolio, see if the lines are smooth and connect at the right spots.

Blowouts

A blowout occurs when the lining needle goes in the skin at the wrong angle and possibly too deep. It commonly happens on a bony area like the collar bone or the shin. Blowouts look like the line in the skin has "blown out" to the side of the intended line, usually on the outside of a curve. It almost looks like the line has a shadow.

Blowouts can disappear over time. Bad blowouts can make the line look quite wide and can heal into a scar at the point of entry. Usually the tattooist will cover them with some black shading. Blowouts can happen to any tattooist while he or she is tattooing over certain areas of the body, but they are still considered kind of embarrassing. If you see a constant amount of obvious blowouts in a tattooist's work, you may want to find someone else. One blowout here or there is forgivable, especially in a large tattoo like a rib panel, but too many means more experience is needed.

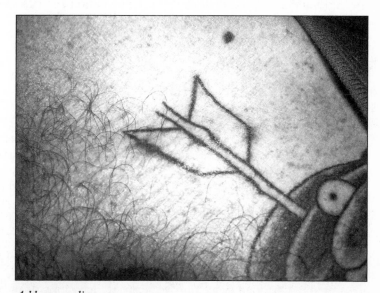

A blown outline.

Not Deep Enough

An inexperienced tattooist may not have the confidence to really get the line in deep enough to stay. As we have gone over previously, the line work is the frame of the tattoo. If you have a weak outline, you have a weak tattoo.

A weak line will appear faded and scratchy. On close examination, you will be able to see the individual marks from each pin in the tattoo needle. It will look like a bunch of tiny thin lines as opposed to one solid line. On really stretchy parts of the body like the stomach, this is common. An experienced tattooist will either get it done once or just do one more pass to make sure the line is in there.

Too Deep

Getting a tattoo that is too deep can be very painful. Such a tattoo will also cause excessive damage to your skin and cause the entire area to be much more sore than it should be. The next day it will feel like someone hit you with a bat. Also, the ink in the tattoo will either fall out, scar up, or heal in a very blurry way. Usually it's a combination of all three. The best way to avoid this situation is to choose your tattooist after seeing healed work first hand or photographs of work that has healed properly.

Coloring and Shading

The majority of your tattoo will most likely be made up of coloring and shading. That is, coloring and shading will take up the most surface area of the tattoo. As we went over in Chapter 5, traditionally the coloring and shading are done with a mag. For your average tattoo, the black and or gray shading will be done first, and then the color will be placed on top of that if the design calls for color.

We know tattooing can be uncomfortable. It's nice to only have a tattoo done once. Some colors will appear brighter if they are layered or tattooed twice on two separate occasions. It means more pigment in the skin, which makes for an extra-solid tattoo. Most of the time and with most tattoos, just once is enough.

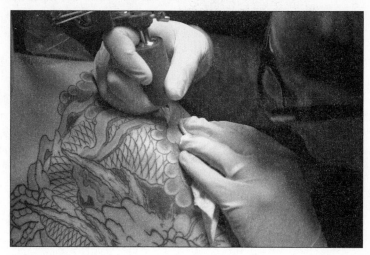

Shading being added.

Looking closely at the coloring and shading of a tattoo, you can tell if the tattooist will do a good job. You will see if artistically she can make your tattoo attractive or will leave you with a large, lumpy scab that takes months to heal. The artistic sense of the tattooist can make or break your tattoo.

Solid

To keep from having to go back for a touch-up that isn't your fault, look to see if the tattoos in the portfolio are solid. Make sure the tattooist has shaded all the way up to the line. You shouldn't be able to see any patches of skin popping through. All those little nooks and crannies and dips and curves should be filled in accordingly.

Depending on the style of the tattoo, the black shading should appear relatively smooth and even. You don't want it to look scratchy and careless. Some traditional sailor tattoos are purpose-fully done with rough black shading—you can see the marks of the shader—to make them appear as if they were done by an old-timer, as well as to make them look tough, like it hurt.

A high-quality tattoo. Tattooed by John Reardon.

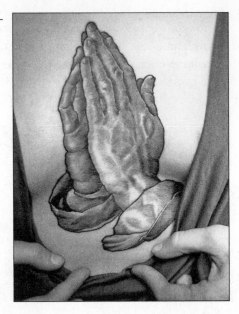

Gray shading should be smooth and solid, as well. It shouldn't appear splotchy or vary too much. Bad shading on a portrait will look horrible. Some tattooists specialize in black and gray realistic tattoos. If you want one of those tattoos, search out an expert.

Chewed and Scarred

One of the major points to this book is to keep you from getting a tattoo that is chewed and scarred. It happens all the time. So many tattooists just don't really know what they are doing, and so many shop owners don't tattoo so they have no idea that their tattooists are messing people up. To them, it is all about the money. Get them in and get them out before they know what happened.

Getting a tattoo that is really scarred can happen from the tattooist overworking the skin. He spends too much time tattooing one area, so the skin then becomes chewed and will heal into a scar. Many tattooists with years of experience know how to overwork an area of the tattoo without causing too much damage to the skin. This enables them to make smooth color blends, smooth transitions from black to color, and add highlights.

You can tell the skin has been chewed by looking at the texture of it. You should be able to see the skin's natural texture as if nothing had happened. Your skin should just be bleeding a bit and be a new color. When the skin has been overworked, it will start to look like ground hamburger. It won't feel good, either, and will probably be bleeding profusely.

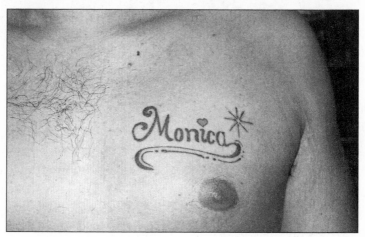

A poor-quality tattoo.

Inkformation

As mentioned in previous chapters, how well you take care of your tattoo will determine how it heals. If you allow it to form thick scabs from over-moisturizing it or letting it dry out, you may cause the ink to fall out. Picking the scabs may cause the tattoo to scar. Letting the fresh tattoo sit in the sun will also cause a bad reaction. Your skin needs time to heal, so take care of your tattoo. Your tattooist will be able to tell if you didn't take care of the tattoo and might not fix it for you, or might charge you to fix it.

Is It Bright or Faded?

In Chapter 5, we went over the different inks tattooists use. We learned that tattooists use many different brands. Some ink is much better than others. A good ink will heal looking more vibrant than a bad ink, no matter how good the tattooist is. The ink will determine the intensity of your tattoo.

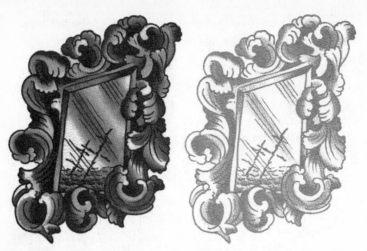

The tattoo should be bold not weak or faded. Design by Dan Trocchio.

Luckily, if you find a good, experienced tattooist, chances are he will have some of the best ink to use. The best way to tell if the tattooist's ink is good is by seeing a healed tattoo he has done. It is better to see an older tattoo to really gauge the lasting quality of the ink. For many people, it isn't possible to see an aged tattoo, so you might just have to settle for the photos in a portfolio.

A recently done tattoo should appear to be very bright. The ink is still close to the surface of the skin, as we learned in Chapter 4. If the color in the tattoo looks really light or faded, the ink may not have gone in deep enough. The black should look black, not gray-ish. Usually if the color is splotchy or faded, you will also notice that the line work is lame as well. Technical problems due to inexperience or poor ability usually come hand in hand.

Too Light/Too Dark

Making sure that a tattooist is technically capable and confident is the first step to finding your tattooist. If you are just getting something small or you simply want to get a piece of flash from the wall, you are all set. As we have learned, there are many great tattooists who only tattoo flash designs, and they probably do them better than any tattooist who prefers to draw custom tattoos.

Picking out a tattooist to do a custom tattoo when you don't have a fully rendered design in front of you can be tricky.

For a custom tattoo, you want to make sure the outcome will be well balanced. You have already taken a look at the drawing ability of the tattooist, but now you need to make sure she can choose the right colors. You want to make sure that she will use the right amount of black so the tattoo will be in good balance.

When looking at portfolios, you will want to observe the tattooist's color work. Make sure the colors she chooses aren't too gaudy and don't clash unless that's what you are looking for. This becomes an issue of personal style. If you like the colors the tattooist uses in her tattoos and how she combines them, you have found yourself a winner.

Tattoos need a certain amount of black to make the colors bright. It's the contrast that pushes out the color, making it vibrant. If a tattooist doesn't put enough black in a tattoo, it won't look as bright. You will see this more as the tattoo ages over the years. Tattoos with only color tend to get very blurry and weak with time. They may look great for a while, but not forever.

A tattoo with too much black will appear too dark and may end up looking like a black blob as the years go by. Some people prefer to have very dark tattoos. Dark tattoos can have an eerie or mysterious feel. They can also look masculine; so ladies, if you want a feminine feel to your tattoo, don't let your tattoist overdo it on the black. Let him know in the first place before it's too late.

An example of a dark flash. Design by John Reardon

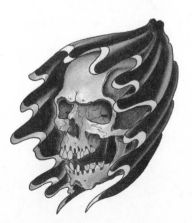

Be sure to fully examine the portfolio of the tattooist you are getting your tattoo from. You don't want to make a mistake by letting yourself get butchered. You will just have to find someone else to fix it and spend more money. Take your time with this process. It will save you a lot of time and money as well as keep you from having a huge headache.

The Least You Need to Know

- ◆ The best way to find a good tattooist is to look through tattooists' portfolios.

- ◆ Presentation is not as important as the work itself when evaluating a portfolio.

- ◆ High-quality photos, originality, and good line work are the things to look for in a portfolio.

- ◆ Shaky lines and blowouts are a sign of an inexperienced or poor tattooist.

- ◆ Shading and strong outlines are important aspects of finished tattoos.

Part 3

Get in the Chair

Now you're ready to start the actual process of getting a tattoo. You know where you are going to get the tattoo and who is going to do the tattoo. All you have to do now is go and get it.

Before you go running into the tattoo shop, we'll go over a few things first. This part is designed to show you who and what you will encounter. You will see what the actual tattoo process consists of as well as how to take care of your tattoo.

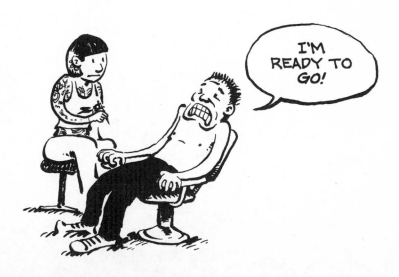

I'M READY TO GO!

Chapter 10

Self-Preparation

In This Chapter

- ◆ The importance of eating
- ◆ Being physically ready
- ◆ Things not to do before getting tattooed
- ◆ What to bring with you

Life seems to go much easier when you are prepared. It is just easier to get things done that way. It's the same with getting a tattoo. You could just walk into a random tattoo shop and pick something off of the wall without any preparation. What if the tattooist doesn't know what he is doing? What if you can't sit there during the tattoo because you are hungry and too tired? You will want to be ready when the needle is coming at you.

There are a few basic things to know that can help you have a comfortable tattoo experience. Getting a tattoo is really very simple as long as you follow these basic steps. In this chapter we will take a look at what you can do to prepare yourself to make your tattoo go smoothly, and a few things that you may want to avoid so you won't be asked to come back to the shop another time.

Eat!

We all need to eat. Hunger can make any situation more difficult than it needs to be. A tattoo can be a big step for you. A good meal is a great way to celebrate this new change in your life. It can help put you in a good mood, so treat yourself so that you are more positive for your tattoo. Having food in your stomach is a good idea when you get tattooed. Let's take a closer look at the benefits of eating as well as why you need to eat.

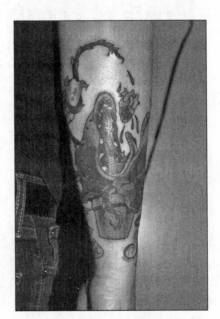

You should always eat before getting a tattoo. Tattoo by Eli Quinters.

Why You Should Eat

It is important to eat at least three hours before getting a tattoo. It is not uncommon for the tattooist or floor person to ask you if you have eaten in the last three hours and tell you to come back after you have had something to eat. Eating a decent-sized meal before getting a tattoo will help you relax during the tattoo process. You will want to be as relaxed as possible, and it's a good excuse to eat some good food.

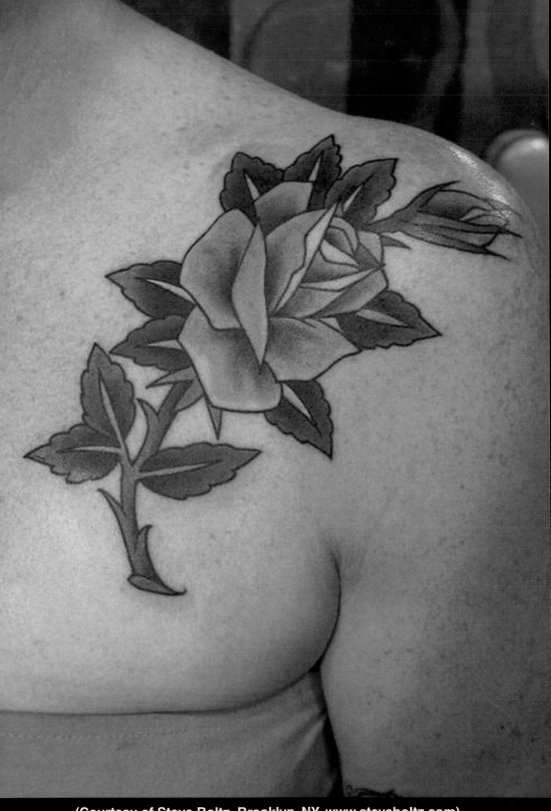

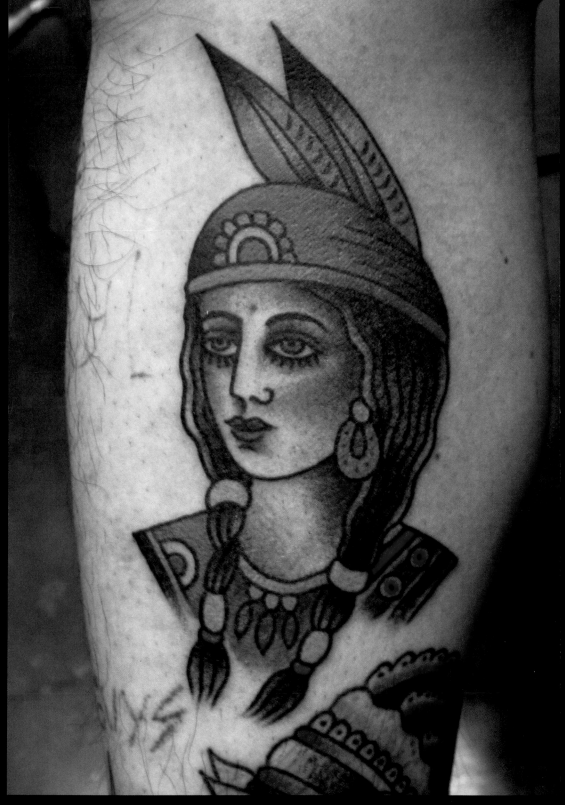

(Courtesy of Steve Boltz, Brooklyn, NY, www.steveboltz.com)

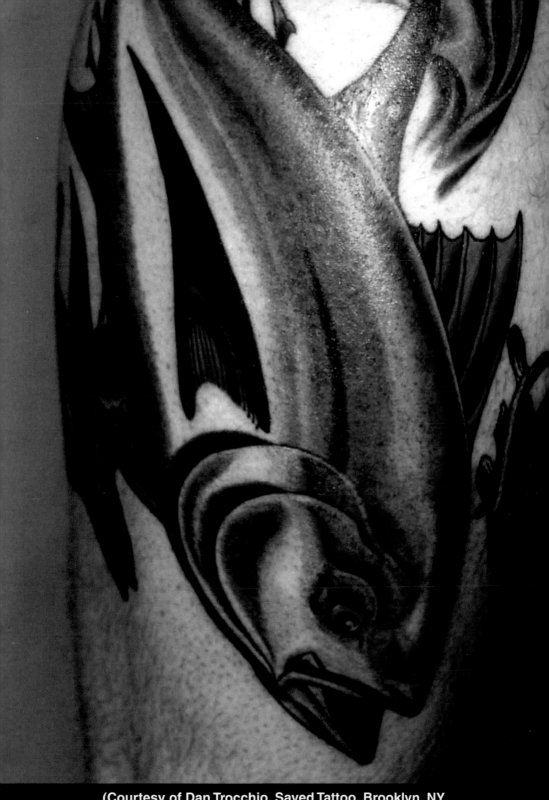

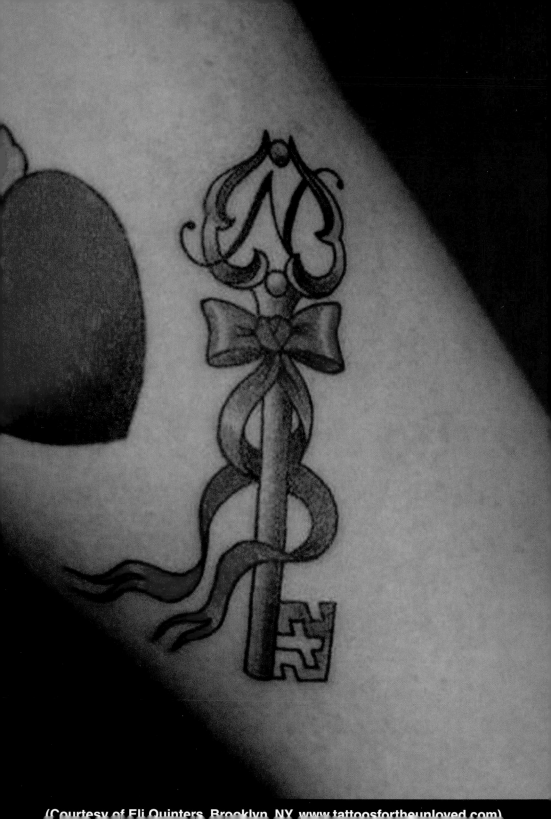

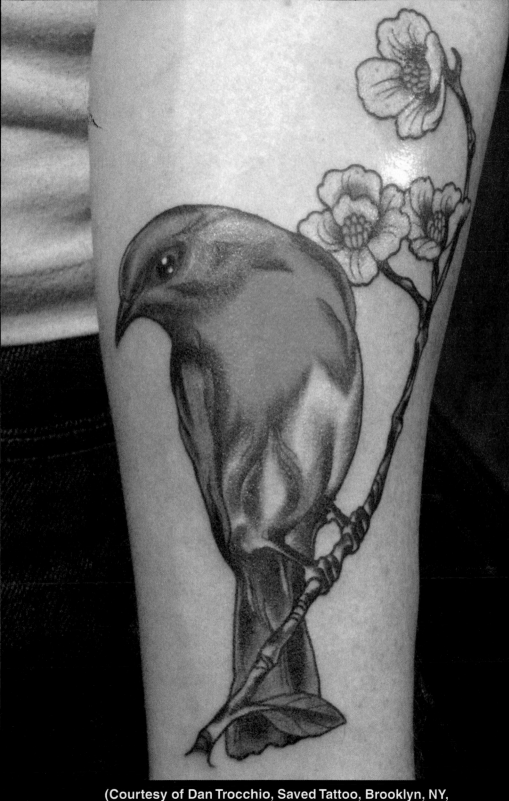

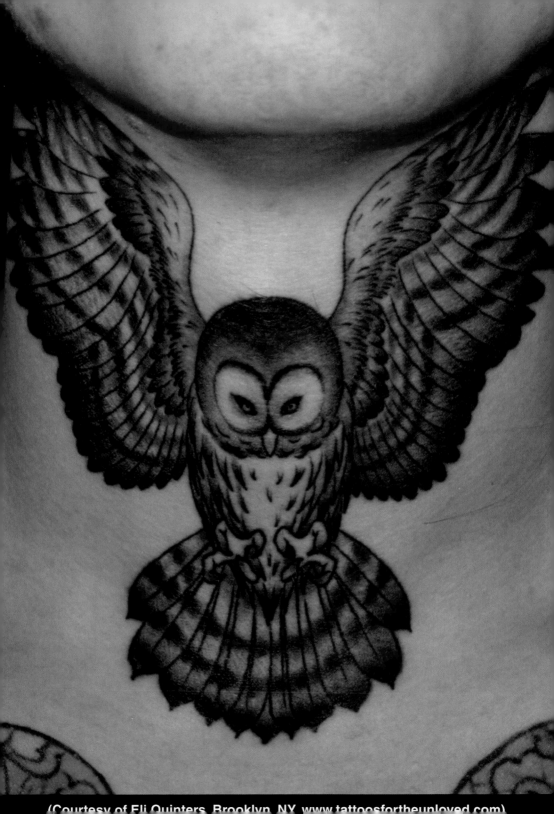

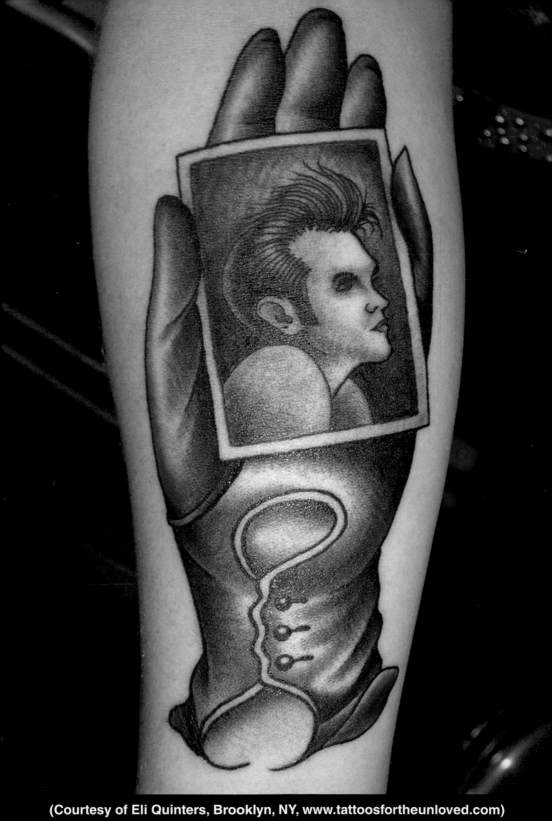

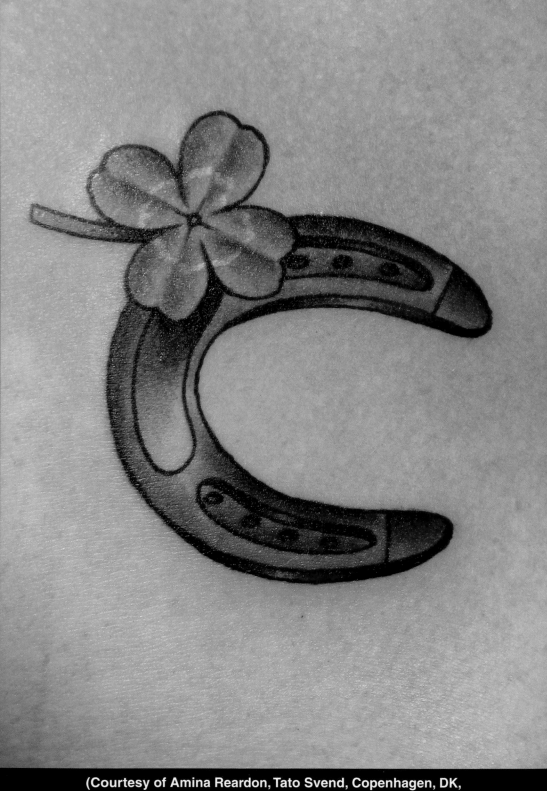

(Courtesy of Amina Reardon, Tato Svend, Copenhagen, DK,
www.aminareardontattoos.com)

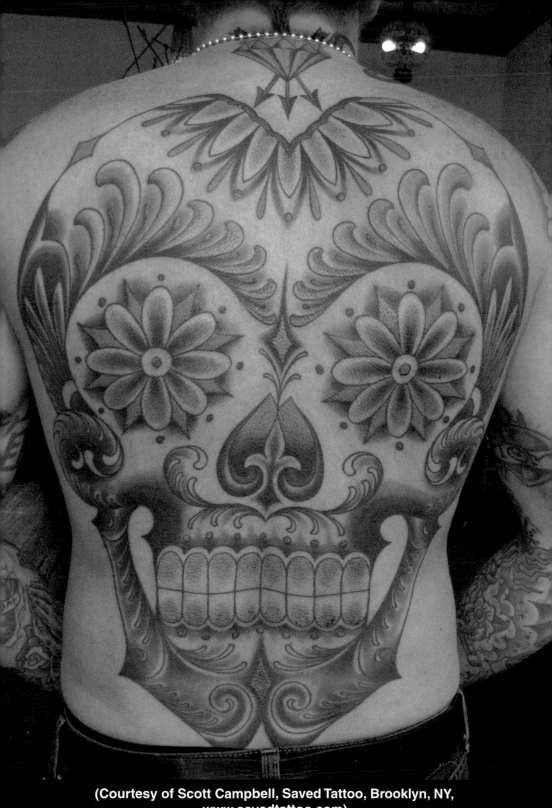

(Courtesy of Scott Campbell, Saved Tattoo, Brooklyn, NY,
www.savedtattoo.com)

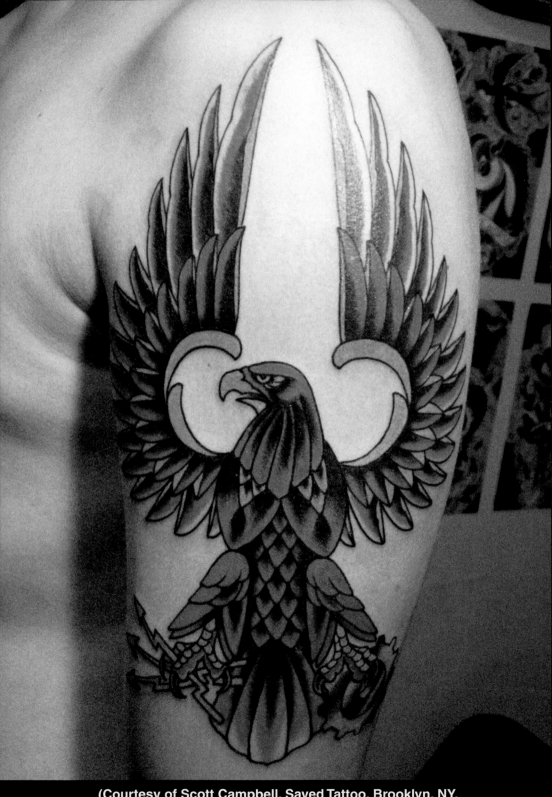

(Courtesy of Scott Campbell, Saved Tattoo, Brooklyn, NY,
www.savedtattoo.com)

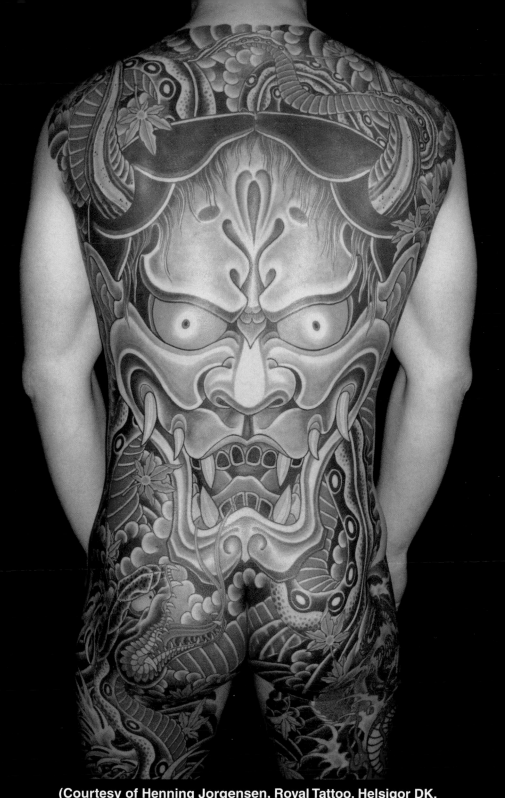

(Courtesy of Henning Jorgensen, Royal Tattoo, Helsigor DK,
www.royaltattoo.com)

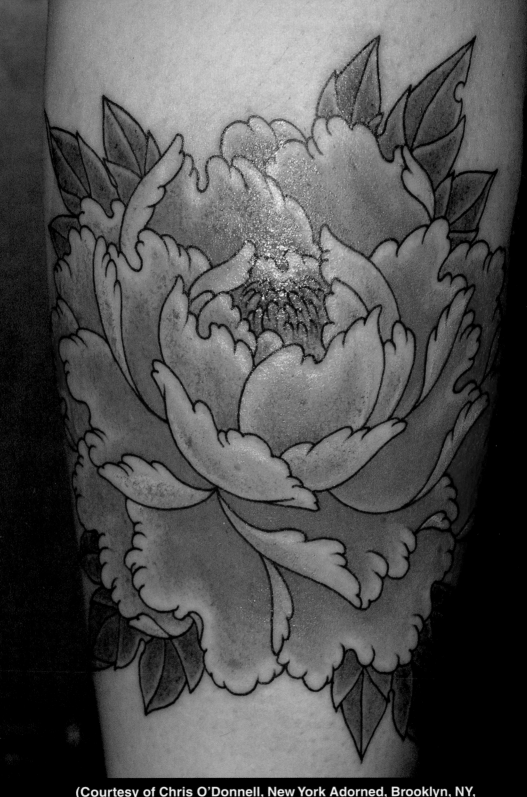

(Courtesy of Chris O'Donnell, New York Adorned, Brooklyn, NY,
www.codnyc.com)

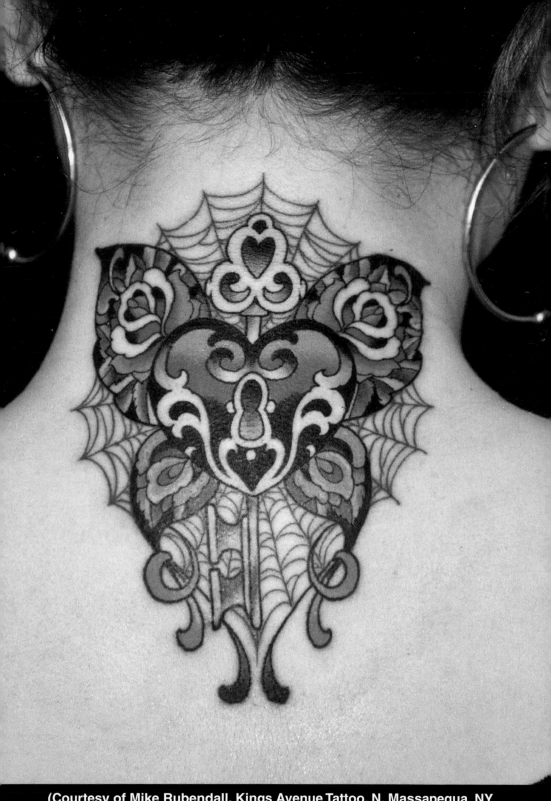

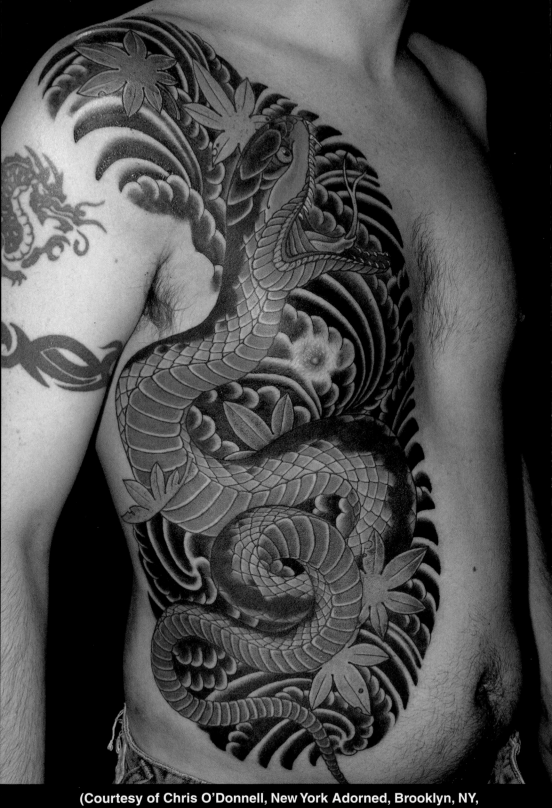

(Courtesy of Chris O'Donnell, New York Adorned, Brooklyn, NY,
www.codnyc.com)

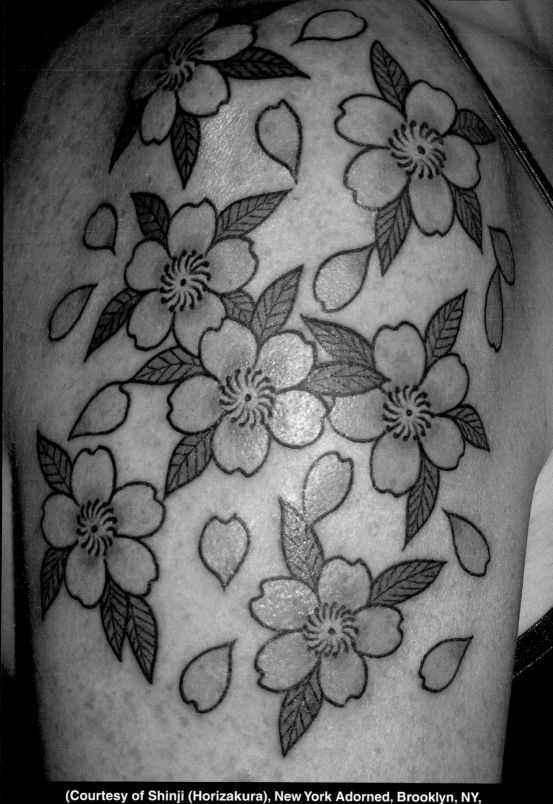

(Courtesy of Shinji (Horizakura), New York Adorned, Brooklyn, NY,
www.nyadorned.com)

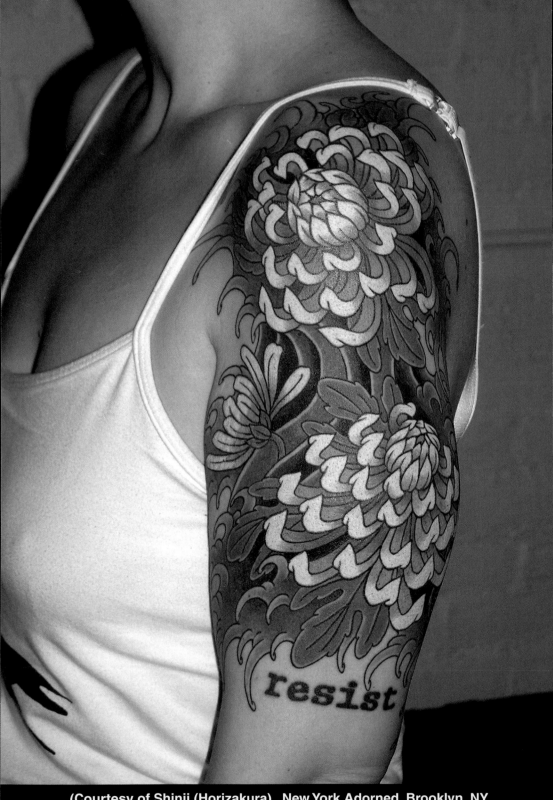

(Courtesy of Shinji (Horizakura) , New York Adorned, Brooklyn, NY,
www.nyadorned.com)

If you try to get tattooed on an empty stomach, you may find that it is hard to concentrate. You will find it hard to sit still so the tattooist can do his job. It is uncomfortable enough getting a tattoo, let alone sitting there with a growling stomach. If your blood-sugar level is down, you also run a higher risk of passing out during the tattoo. Nobody likes passing out during a tattoo.

It is better to eat before you go to the shop. If you are getting a tattoo that will take a few hours, you will definitely want to plan ahead. You won't want to stop mid-tattoo to get something to eat. Also, some tattoo shops are located far away from any fast food. Ordering delivery will take too much time, as you may be finished by the time the food gets there.

When planning what to eat before you get your tattoo, you will want to keep in mind the various reactions you have to different foods. The point of eating before getting a tattoo is so that you will be more comfortable and will be able to relax. You will want to think before you eat. For example, stay away from any food that will give you gas or heartburn. Beans may be your comfort food but those around you won't be comfortable. Trying new foods may be risky, too, as you don't know how your system will react. An emergency run to the bathroom during a tattoo can be a little embarrassing. Also, stay away from foods loaded with sugar. You will need to sit still, and too much sugar may make you antsy.

Flash Tip

For longer tattoo sessions, you may want to bring a small snack like a candy bar, just in case you get a little hungry.

No Caffeine!

Coffee is a very popular beverage among tattooists. It can help them to wake up and to keep tattooing. It is not, however, a good beverage to have before getting a tattoo. Caffeine will most likely make you jumpy. As the tattoo process goes on for longer periods of time, it can become more difficult to sit still. Caffeine will only make that worse.

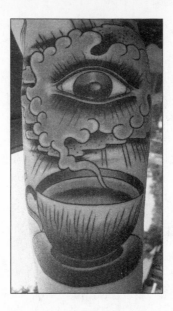

Coffee may taste good, but it doesn't help you to get tattooed. Tattoo by Steve Byrne.

Try drinking something that is caffeine-free. Chamomile tea is good for getting tattooed, as it can make you feel more relaxed. Natural juices that aren't overloaded with sugar are good. Water is the best thing to drink, as there isn't anything in there to make you jumpy.

Be Hydrated

Being dehydrated during a tattoo can be very uncomfortable. It can keep you from ignoring the pain just like being hungry. It's good to drink a good amount of water while you are getting tattooed. Water is easy to clean if you spill it, so many shops will allow you to have it at the tattoo station. But try to not drink too much, or you might need frequent bathroom breaks.

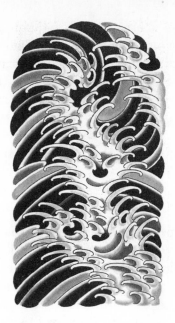

Being dehydrated can make you very uncomfortable when getting tattooed.

Be Well Rested

Being tired when you get a tattoo can make you more susceptible to the pain. You will find it very hard to sit still. As you know, being tired or exhausted can make you grumpy and irritable. That is not how you want to be while sitting under the needle. Getting tattooed can make it worse, and it may make you want to stop or be miserable toward your friends or your tattooist.

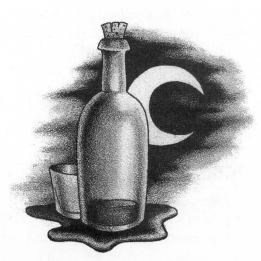

Try to avoid one of these nights before you get tattooed. Design by Eli Quinters, www. tattoosfortheunloved.com.

You may want to plan to have an early night on the eve of getting a large tattoo. Going on a bender the night before your appointment can really make for a bad experience. Getting tattooed with a hangover is not fun at all. You may end up getting sick, which is never a good time. Also, sitting there with a buzzing machine in your ear while your head aches can make the tattoo process seem to last forever. Try to plan ahead so that you are ready to be in the shop for your appointment instead of at home, sick in bed.

Be Clean

Tattooing is an intimate and sterile process. You will want to be clean for the tattoo so you won't run the risk of infection. Tattoo shops put a lot of effort into being a safe and sterile environment for your safety. It doesn't make much sense to jeopardize that by bringing some unnecessary filth into the situation. As you saw in Chapter 8, you expect that the tattooist comes to work nice and fresh everyday so you won't have to deal with something funky while getting tattooed. Likewise, coming straight to the tattoo shop from the construction site or aerobics class may not be such a great idea.

> **Flash Tip**
>
> If you are going to get the top of your foot tattooed, and you think that your feet smell, don't be afraid to go wash your feet in the bathroom. The tattooist will thank you for it.

On the opposite end of the spectrum, overdosing on perfume or deodorant can have a negative consequence, too. You will want the tattooist to take the correct amount of time with your tattoo no matter what the size. You don't want him to rush because he can't breathe. Replacing a shower with an extra dose of cologne is a popular thing to do, but it really just makes the situation worse. Try to relax and plan ahead to get it all done right the first time.

No Drugs, No Alcohol

In the United States, it is illegal to get tattooed while you are under the influence. Some shops will turn you away if they think you have been drinking. The reason for this is to protect you.

They are protecting you from making a bad choice that you might live to regret. Many people get "liquid courage" after a few drinks and think they can do anything. Permanent decisions are better made while sober.

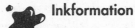 **Inkformation**

Despite popular belief, you have to consume many alcoholic beverages before your blood gets too thinned out for you to get tattooed.

Another reason why drunks are turned away is that they can be very loud and obnoxious. They can make it uncomfortable for other people who are getting tattooed in the shop. This also guards against those who have quick personality changes and get violent or just rude and angry. Drunks don't have the sturdiest of legs and may fall down and hurt themselves or someone else in the shop. If you have been drinking, getting a tattoo may make you upchuck, which can make for a nasty situation.

You must also stay away from drugs when getting a tattoo. Marijuana will make the feeling of the tattoo hurt much more than if you are sober. Although painkillers are legally given for cosmetic surgery, it is still uncertain if you can legally get them for getting large tattoos. One reason for this might be that doctors don't make any money from tattoos, unless they are removing them. However, receiving painkillers to ease the pain of tattooing seems fair, considering that most cosmetic surgery is along the same line of vanity as tattooing. Access to prescription painkillers for getting tattooed is something to keep an eye on, as getting a large tattoo on the ribs can be very difficult to deal with.

Spray Tan

If you know you are going to get a tattoo in the near future, stay away from self-tanning products. There are many physical reasons to stay away from fake tans when you want a tattoo. Your skin will have a different texture, which makes it difficult to tattoo. The stencil will wipe away much faster than normal, leaving the tattooist guessing on what to tattoo, and this may mess up your design.

The chemicals in self-tanners may keep your tattoo from healing properly. You will want your skin to be as clean and natural as it can be when you get your tattoo. It will help the outcome of the tattoo.

No Sunburns

Stay out of the sun before and after you get a tattoo. Sunburned skin is already irritated and trying to heal itself. If you try to get a tattoo on a sunburn, your tattoo may not heal well and you may need to return for touch-ups.

Your skin will already be very sensitive. Getting a tattoo on sensitive skin will hurt much more than normal. Also, a tattooist needs to wipe the area with a paper towel to absorb the excess ink and what little blood comes out. This will be hard to deal with if the entire area is burning in the first place. You can't get a tattoo over blisters, either.

Flash Tip

Sunburned skin is damaged skin and adding a tattoo to the damaged skin can only exacerbate the situation.

After a sunburn heals, the dead skin will peel off like a shedding lizard's. This dead skin can cause a huge headache for your tattooist during a tattoo. If the skin isn't noticeably peeling, the dead skin will still wipe away. It will take with it the stencil or marker the tattooist needs to outline your tattoo. It will make a huge mess of your tattoo. The dead skin will also absorb the ink and make it more difficult for your tattooist to see what he or she is doing. Try to stay out of the sun when you have the itch to get a tattoo.

Leave Your Problems at Home

You can't avoid having problems. That's the way things go. Sometimes these problems can make you want to vent by getting a tattoo. The slight pain can be therapeutic as it forces you to think about the tattoo pain and not your other difficulties. It can really clear your head for a short period of time, which may help you get some balance.

When getting your tattoo, if you let these outside difficulties into the tattoo shop, it may impair your ability to choose a design that you will be happy with for the rest of your life. You don't want to end up with a severed-head tattoo after a breakup with your significant other. If your head is too clouded, come back another time when you can make the right decision.

Physically bringing your problems to the shop, as in bringing the person you are at odds with into the tattoo shop, isn't the best thing to do, either. Tattoo shops are not large places, so any arguing is very noticeable. You may be asked to come back later if you disturb the other clients or distract the tattooist. It will be easier for you to concentrate and sit still during the tattoo if your problems aren't staring you in the face. It's better for everyone if you come to the tattoo shop without any baggage.

Children

A tattoo shop is not a very good place to bring your children. Tattoo shops will often harbor adult-oriented conversations that most parents would not want their kids to hear. Tattooists are also known for having potty mouths. If the shop does piercing, there may be photos of genitals with piercings out in the open for all to see. You may be exposing your children to new things that you may not think they are ready for. Many tattooists have kids, so they can understand the troubles of having them in the shop.

Younger children have a tendency to cry and scream, which can disrupt the entire shop and make it difficult for other clients to get their tattoos in peace. You may be asked to leave and come back without the kids. Many young children don't understand what's happening, and they will start to cry if they think their mommy or daddy is being hurt. Also, small children may try to climb on you or accidentally bump into you while you are getting tattooed. You may end up with a few mistakes in your tattoo, which may not make for a good day in the end.

Most shops are rather strict about not allowing anyone under the age of 18 in the shop. You are better off leaving the kids at home, because most likely they will get bored after the first five minutes anyway.

Bring a Buddy

For your first tattoo, you may want to bring a friend along for moral support. She can give you her opinion and help you make your decisions about what to get tattooed and who to do the tattoo for you. It's nice to have a little backup. Try to bring a friend and not a significant other. Oftentimes significant others will become overbearing and possessive of you. This can lead to your not getting exactly what you want, like his name or a tattoo that he would get instead of a design you were thinking of in the first place. Lovers have a way of doing that.

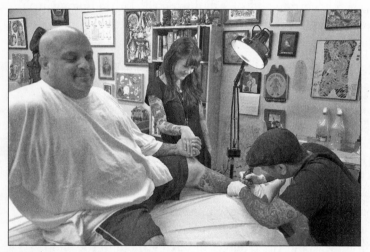

A good friend can be a great comfort while you are getting tattooed.

A good friend is nice to have with you during the tattoo, if it is possible. He can hold your hand if you are nervous or if the tattoo is more sensitive or more difficult to deal with than you thought. It's nice to have him there to get you things, like water or a magazine, when you can't get up during the tattoo. Talking with a good friend can help the time go by faster and make your experience much more pleasant.

Personal Music Player

If you don't want to bring a friend with you or talk to anyone during your tattoo, you can always bring a personal music player like an iPod. Most shops will already have music playing, but it may be something you don't particularly care for. It's easier to have your music to make you feel more comfortable.

Many shops nowadays are starting to have TVs in the tattoo area. TV is great to watch while you are getting tattooed as long as you are into the program. TV makes the time go by much faster. With the advent of small portable movie players like the PSP, video iPods, and iPhones, you can watch whatever you want as long as you have earphones.

Portable video games may work to help pass the time, as well. If you can play a portable video game without moving around too much, you are in business. Just don't move while you are getting tattooed or you may mess up your tattoo.

Tattoo Taboo

Small electronic devices may be distracting for the tattooist, so you may want to ask if it's okay to use one before you turn it on.

Something to Read

Some people like to read while they get tattooed. They find it helps to focus their minds on something other than the feeling of getting tattooed and also helps pass the time. Magazines are good to have because during the tattoo it may be difficult to focus on reading but you can still look at the pictures. Most shops will have stacks of tattoo magazines so you can look for your next idea.

You may find reading a little difficult to do during a tattoo. This depends on the placement of the tattoo. If you are getting tattooed on your arm, you won't be able to flip the page. If you are getting your chest tattooed, your book will get in the way of the tattooist, as his head will be right next to yours. Newspapers can take up too much space and a heavy book may be too large to hold. It is up to you to figure out what you will need or want to keep you entertained during the tattoo. Many clients simply prefer to sit, relax, and meditate to help them through the tattoo process.

Reading may help you pass the time.

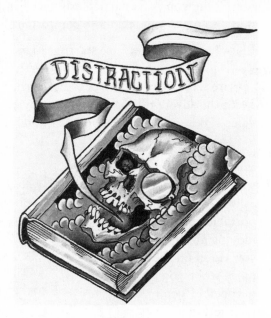

The Least You Need to Know

- A good meal before a tattoo will help you relax.

- Being well rested for your tattoo will make it easier for you to get tattooed.

- You cannot legally get a tattoo while you are under the influence.

- Your skin has to be healthy in order to get a tattoo.

- You may want to bring someone or something to help you pass the time while you are being tattooed.

Chapter 11

The Shop

In This Chapter

◆ What to expect when you walk into a shop

◆ Here is where you get your tattoo

◆ Meeting the people who will help you

◆ The different people in the shop

The tattoo shop is the heart of tattooing—it is here where the business starts. It is here where a tattooist can have a base to set up and build a career. It is a house of pain and pleasure, and, of course, a lot of coffee drinking.

Tattoo shops are really very simple places. You will use them to help you find your tattooist and your design. They are set up to run specifically to help you get your tattoo. Let's take a deeper look at what you will find in a tattoo shop, so you will know who and what to expect.

Shop Set-Up

There is a basic layout that every tattoo shop will follow. This layout makes the tattoo shop run in an efficient and practical way. It enables you to feel comfortable when you walk in to check out the shop, and for you to feel comfortable while you are getting tattooed. There are three basic parts needed to run a tattoo shop: the front room or waiting room, the tattoo station, and the sterilization area.

Front/Waiting Room

The first room you will walk into in a tattoo shop is the front room or waiting room. It's very much like a doctor's office but with more style. Every shop is different, so every waiting room will have a different flavor to it. Some shops put a lot of effort into decorating the waiting room with paintings and specialized furniture or designs painted on the floor. This is where most of the customizing in the shop is done, as the rest of the shop needs to be more practical. You will be able to tell the overall style of the shop by the waiting room.

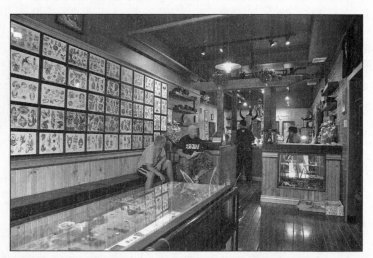

The front waiting area with flash mounted on the wall. (Hold Fast Tattoo, Brooklyn, NY).

Here you will have your first encounter with either a floor person or a tattooist. The waiting room or front room is, in a sense, a greeting room for you. There will usually be couches or chairs for you to sit on while you wait or look through the portfolios. Nowadays, most shops are starting to use wireless Internet, so if you have a laptop you can surf the Internet while you wait.

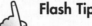

Flash Tip

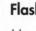

When you walk into a shop and there is no one to be seen, start shuffling through the portfolios or flash. Someone will hear you and come running to help you out.

Most shops will not allow customers to bring food into the waiting room. It is mainly a cleanliness issue. It's not a good idea to have a front waiting room of a tattoo shop smelling like fast food. It would make the shop seem like an unclean and unsafe place to get a tattoo. Usually a drink with a closed lid is fine. You will want to drink some water while you are getting tattooed, anyway; getting tattooed makes you kind of thirsty.

Flash Locations

The front room or waiting area is where you will find the flash. Many shops will have all the flash in a rack attached to the wall. This way more than one person can look through it at once. Flash can also be mounted on the wall like wallpaper. This is a good effect because you can stand in one position and examine the different designs without anyone getting in your way.

Flash Tip

Many tattooists will have flash that they have made in the shop's collection of flash. It is another way you can see what their work looks like.

Shops will generally have lots of flash for you to choose from. Many shops will have so much that they have to keep the extra flash in books. These are usually located within view on a table or desk in the room. They are usually labeled with the contents, so you can easily find what you are looking for. In more custom shops, where the tattooists prefer to draw tattoos, they will often still have some flash kept in a flash book.

For pricing of the different designs, some shops have developed a system of numbering and lettering, which will enable you to figure out how much your tattoo will cost without having to talk to someone. This works best if you are in a very busy shop and the tattooists are overwhelmed. Usually there is a chart on the shop wall that explains how to price tattoos. However, many shops still rely on pricing each tattoo individually. When that is the case, you will need to speak to someone about pricing.

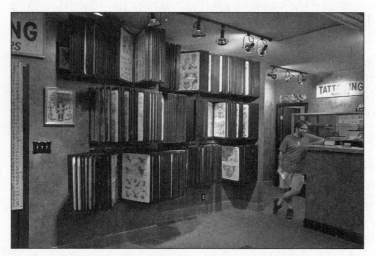

An example of a flash rack like you will find in most shops. (Flyrite Tattoo, Brooklyn, NY).

As the computer era is slowly coming of age in the tattoo shop, computers have begun to take the place of flash racks and flash books. This is a great system, as it enables you to search through numerous designs, many more than a shop could fit on the wall. Another advantage is that when you have made your selection, the tattooist can probably print it out, saving time on setting up.

Portfolios

As we have seen throughout the book, portfolios are the representation of each tattooist. These are generally kept in the front waiting room. They should be somewhere very noticeable such as at a front desk or coffee table. Sometimes a shop will keep them behind the front desk and only take them out when asked to. This usually occurs in a very busy shop where clients don't ask to see the portfolios or if the shop has had a portfolio stolen in the past.

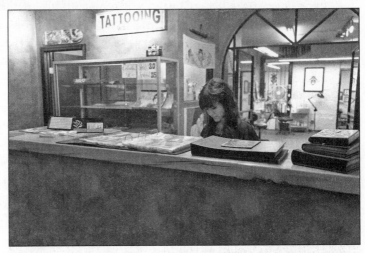

A front desk with portfolios. (Flyrite Tattoo, Brooklyn, NY).

As with the flash designs, some shops are now using computer screens to showcase the different tattooists' portfolios. With a computer, you can take a look at the different artists' work without having to wait for someone else to finish a certain portfolio. It can make it a little more convenient for everyone involved in the process.

Tattoo Station

The tattoo station is where the magic happens. This is where you will be tattooed. Tattoo stations will differ from tattooist to tattooist and from shop to shop. Some tattoo stations are set up so that they each consist of a separate individual room. This is nice for privacy and can make it easier to concentrate when you are getting tattooed. Many shops are set up with individual booths that have about a 4-foot-high wall separating each other. This provides separation but still allows for airflow and the ability to see who is coming in and out of the shop. A popular and easy way to set up a shop is to place stations around a large, open room. You will be able to see what other people are getting tattooed as well as possibly spark up a conversation with a fellow client.

The tattoo stations may be set up differently but they all have the same basic ingredients. There will sometimes be a sink nearby for easy access to water. The tattooists will keep their machines here as well as all the other necessary tools of the trade that you saw in Chapter 5. You may be able to see some drawings taped to the wall that the tattooist has drawn for other customers' tattoos or just for fun.

A tattoo station will usually have at least two chairs, usually with wheels on the bottom to allow for easy maneuvering during the tattoo. Some shops like to have the client sit in a barber's chair or a dentist's chair. These chairs can be adjusted to fit the situation of the tattoo. A massage table will also be near, just in case you need to lie down for the tattoo.

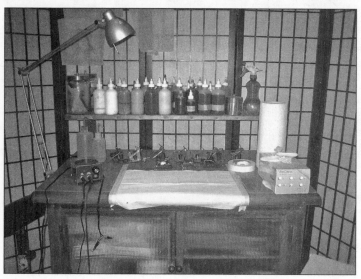

One of the tattoo stations at Saved Tattoo, Brooklyn, NY.

Many tattooists will decorate their station with different kinds of collections. You may find yourself staring at a Star Wars figure collection or a Todd McFarlane figure collection. Many tattooists will collect paintings or prints from other tattooists and hang them by their station. In addition, most tattooists will have a large collection of reference books.

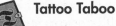

Tattoo Taboo

Due to possible contamination of the equipment, it is a good idea to not touch anything in the tattoo station unless you are asked to.

With all this stuff by the station, there may not be enough room for more than one friend to watch you get tattooed. With all the action of a busy shop, sometimes there isn't even enough room for that person. Don't worry, though; getting tattooed is not that bad, especially if it's your first one.

Drawing Room or Back Room

In many shops, there will be a back room or drawing room that may be off-limits to the customer. Drawing a tattoo design can take a lot of concentration, so it's important to let the artists do their thing uninterrupted. Some tattooists will have you stay there to check out how the drawing is coming along, or to help guide them to make the process go faster. Drawing rooms will usually have a small reference library to help the tattooist get the job done right.

Many times a back room is where the people who work in the shop eat their various meals of the day. Some shops will have a small refrigerator, coffee machine, or water dispenser in the back room. Often the photocopier and stencil machine will be housed there, too, along with the shop computer. All shops run a little differently but they all have the same basic components.

The Sterilization Area

One of the most important parts of the shop is the sterilization area. Without this area, the shop would not be able to clean the equipment and would be shut down. This is where the dirty work is done and then sterilized. Here the shop brings all of its contaminated tools after each use, such as dirty needles and used tubes. The needles are put in the sharps container while the tubes are either placed in a tub of water to soak or in an ultrasonic cleaner.

There will always be a sink in the sterilization area, which will be used to dispose of the water used to clean the tubes in order to change colors during your tattoo. The tubes will also be scrubbed in this sink. Although the sink is sterilized with some form of surface sterilizer such as Matacide, it's a good idea to never use the sink in the sterilization area for other purposes. Even the people who work in the shop always consider this sink contaminated and off-limits to everything but contaminated tattoo equipment.

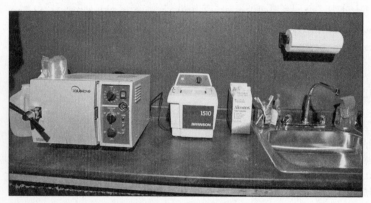

Here is what you would find in a typical sterilization area.

The autoclave will be in the sterilization area, ready to sterilize all the used equipment. In this area are also the supplies needed to run the autoclave such as autoclave bags and distilled water. Sometimes shops will keep all of the other cleaning supplies here, too, such as extra paper towels or gallons of green soap.

Inkformation

You already know smoking is bad for your health, but that doesn't stop smokers from needing a cigarette. The reality is that some people still smoke. In many states in the United States, it is becoming illegal to smoke in public places. Smoking can make a clean place really dingy and smell bad. Most shops won't allow you to smoke inside because they need to stay clean.

Many tattooists smoke, though, so some shops will have a back area where you and your tattooist can have a cigarette. You may have to step out the front door to smoke even if it's raining or freezing. But if you are a smoker, you are probably already used to that.

The People

Tattoo shops generally operate with a very low number of people. Sometimes one tattooist will open up a tattoo shop and run it by himself without the assistance of a floor person or manager. Larger and busier shops will try to support as many tattooists as they can to make more money.

When working with a small number of people, it is easy for lives to intertwine. Often the people working together in a shop will form a kind of family bond. They get to know each other well by sharing their problems and helping each other out. They all want you to get a good tattoo so you will show other people and send more people their way. Let's look at the different people who you will find in a tattoo shop.

Floor Person

The first person who will take care of you in a tattoo shop will be the floor person. He will be the first person you meet. He can help you find what you are looking for and guide you along the way. He will be the medium between you and the tattooist and should be able to answer most of your questions. The floor person is also the one who will set you up with an appointment and take deposits for designs.

A good floor person will also take care of the tattooists in the shop so that the tattooists can put all of their energy into making sure your tattoo is perfect. The floor person will be the one to get things for the tattooists such as coffee or lunch. He can also set up the tattoo station for your tattoo while the tattooist is resting or drawing your tattoo. After the tattoo is complete, a good floor person will clean up the area and reset it for the next tattoo.

It is often the floor person's job to make sure the shop is clean and sterile. He will take care of the bathroom and make sure the floors are mopped daily. The sterilization of the equipment is also part of his job. He will scrub the tubes and make sure the autoclave is running properly.

This all may sound like a lot of work and it is, but don't worry, it comes with benefits. The benefit of being a floor person is usually getting free tattoos. Also, most shops don't open until noon, so they get to sleep in.

Not all tattoo shops have a floor person to take care of the customers. Sometimes the tattooist will have to take care of all of the floor person's duties. It's usually in busier shops that a floor person is needed so that the tattooists can do their jobs without distraction.

Piercer

Some tattoo shops have a piercer. This is the person who takes care of you if you want to get pierced. Some piercers will branch out and do other forms of body modification; it's not all belly buttons and tongues for these piercers. Many will do branding, where the skin is burned with a hot or super-cooled piece of metal or a cauterizer to leave a scar in some design or pattern. The more skilled piercers will do surgical implants, meaning they insert an object under the skin to create a certain shape or design. Many piercers will be part of what are called suspensions. A suspension is the process of inserting hooks into the flesh of specific places on the body in order to be raised up to hang by the hooks. This creates a rush of adrenalin that some people enjoy. Many people find it a very unique experience. For more on the subject, go to www.bmezine.com.

Not all piercers are into all of this body modification. Many piercers will act as the floor person if they aren't busy. It can also be that the floor person just knows how to do small, average piercings like eyebrows and nostrils, and for them, piercing is just for a little cash on the side and to take care of the few customers who come in and want it done.

Apprenticeship

Every tattooist has to start somewhere. The best way for a person to learn how to tattoo properly is to become an apprentice.

An apprenticeship is like college for a tattooist. Not all colleges are great and not everyone can get into every college. It's important for an aspiring tattooist to find a mentor who can teach her all she needs to know, because it will affect her tattoo career in the long run.

An apprentice should be able to draw well and have some form of art background. She must already have started collecting tattoos and continue to get them so she can watch and learn. Learning about the history of tattooing and being interested in what is current in the industry is important as well.

An apprentice will do all the jobs the floor person does, but usually for free. She gets paid through what she is learning. The harder she works, the more she will learn in an ideal situation. In most situations, the apprentice will be tattooed for free so that she can watch and learn. The whole process usually lasts for at least one year before finding a job at another shop or starting to tattoo clients in the shop she learned in.

 Inkformation

Becoming a tattooist is a lifelong commitment, which starts with a proper apprenticeship.

Tattooist

As you already know, the tattooist will be the person tattooing you. He is the whole reason you are there. If there is a really good floor person in the shop, the sole job of the tattooist is to draw and tattoo. If there is no floor person, then the tattooist must clean all of his own equipment and make sure the shop is clean.

A tattooist also needs to take care of advertisement, as far as getting cards and stickers printed. He will often draw all of the propaganda that comes from the shop. T-shirts and bumper stickers usually come from the hands of the tattooist. (Some of them even find time to put together books.) Websites also need to be kept up on, so that you can see the newest tattoos done at the shop.

Inkformation

In every shop, there will be someone just hanging out for fun. For some reason, people like to hang out in tattoo shops. They can be anyone from the guy who delivers food everyday to the shop to a client who gets tattooed there quite often. They are usually very nice, because they don't want to make the tattoo shop lose any business. Often you will be able to see firsthand on these people healed tattoos that have come from the shop.

The Least You Need to Know

◆ The front room or waiting room is where you will be greeted and where you will be able to look through portfolios and the different tattoo designs.

◆ All shops are set up differently and each tattooist will set up their tattoo station to how they work.

◆ Everyone who works at a tattoo shop is their to help you get your tattoo.

◆ You will find all kinds of people can be found hanging out at the shop.

Chapter 12

The Moment of Truth

In This Chapter

- ◆ Preparing your skin
- ◆ Getting your design on properly
- ◆ Perfect positioning for you and your artist
- ◆ Your possible reactions to getting tattooed

You have chosen your design as well as who shall be permanently putting it on your body. You are well fed and quite relaxed. You are ready for the chair! There is no turning back now. You are in it to win it.

Your nerves may be building up in anticipation while you are waiting in the waiting room or even during the car or subway ride to the shop. That is perfectly normal. Soon you will be invited to "sit in the chair." It will still be a few moments before that first initial poke, while your tattooist sets up a few things.

In this chapter, we will go over the process of getting tattooed. You will feel much more comfortable when you know what is going on. A relaxed client is a good client.

Putting on the Stencil

With most one-point tattoos, the artist will use what we call a *stencil*. We use stencils so you can see how the design looks on your body before it is there permanently. A stencil can be used more than once, just in case it needs to be repositioned. Stencils also give tattooists a clear guide to work from. Some artists like to change the design a little while they are tattooing, in order to give the design a more personal touch. This may happen, especially if the design is flash from the wall and the artist has already done that design more than three times that week.

def•i•ni•tion

A **stencil** is a copy of your design, which is usually in outline form. Tattooists use stencils to give you a good idea of what the tattoo will look like on your body before they get started.

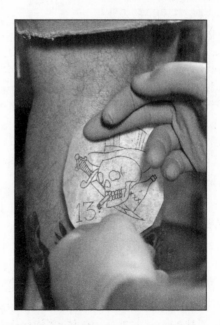

Chops of Hold Fast Tattoo puts the stencil on his client.

Skin Preparation

Before your tattooist puts the stencil on your body, your skin must be properly prepared. To do this, the artist needs four basic things: watered-down soap in a spray or squirt bottle (preferably green soap, a hospital-grade soap, or some form of antibacterial soap), alcohol in a spray-squirt bottle or pad, a razor, and paper towels.

The basic formula for prepping your skin goes like this:

1. Wash the skin. Use soap, scrubbing a bit to get off any dead skin or dirt.

2. Shave hair from the area. More soap may be added to shave the area. Hair harbors bacteria and may also interfere with the stencil. Some tattooists shave dry, without soap, which works just as well. Shaved hair will grow back through the tattoo. Hair will not affect the tattoo at all, but it may cover the tattoo depending on the thickness of the hair.

3. Alcohol is applied to the area as a disinfectant. This may sting a bit, especially if the shaving left a small cut or razor burn, which happens now and again. Sometimes alcohol is applied before the soap, which is also fine.

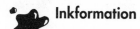

Inkformation

Some artists use iodine to disinfect the skin. Many people are allergic to iodine, so most tattooists just stick with the alcohol disinfectant.

You are sterile and just about ready for the stencil. Now the excitement really begins.

Double-Check

This is the moment to recheck the design to be sure everything is the way you want it. If there are words in the design, now is the time to be absolutely sure of the spelling—it is a good idea to check the words in some form of dictionary. If there isn't a dictionary in the shop, try using an online dictionary.

It can be frustrating for a tattooist to redraw the design after the stencil is on the body. It is one thing to redraw the design so that it better fits the body, because that's part of the job; however, to needlessly go back to the drawing board because the customer wasn't paying attention to his design is wasting time.

Stand Straight

Now it is time to put the stencil on your body. Most of the time, you will need to stand up and stand straight with your arms loosely hanging by your side. For most of the areas of your body, this is the position in which your tattoo must look normal. Remember, when you move, your skin moves along with your tattoo.

Chops is pulling off the stencil paper, and you can see the stencil left on the skin.

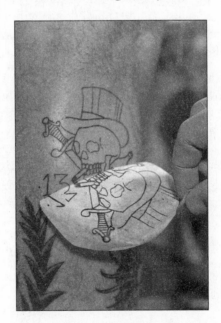

For places such as your underarm, you will stand straight with your arm out, perpendicular to your body.

For forearms it is okay to sit. Here it is important to line up your hand with your elbow in order to place the design in between the two.

A lower leg or foot may entail standing on a chair or stool so the tattooist isn't lying on the ground trying to line up the design with your body.

Artists will have their own way to place the stencil on the body. It is best to let them do what they need to do in order to have a well-placed tattoo.

It is normal for customers to have to undress a bit so their clothing is out of the way. For example, to line up a lower-back tattoo, the top of the customer's butt must be exposed to use as a marker in order to place the stencil in the middle of the back. Most shops will have either private rooms, pull curtains, or folding screens. Tattooists, like doctors, have seen everything, so try to relax. If you feel really uncomfortable, don't be afraid to say so.

One Last Look

After the stencil is placed on your body, it is vital to get a good look at it in the mirror. As amazing as tattoo artists are, they still are human and sometimes need to do stencils a few times before they feel the stencil is ready to be tattooed. Also, you may want the tattoo in a very specific place, which may call for the stencil to be redone a few times before you are satisfied. This happens a lot with symmetrical tattoos or with tattoos that need to line up with another tattoo. Here is a list of things to check while looking to see if your stencil is on correctly:

- ◆ Is it straight up and down or in the middle?
- ◆ Is it placed where you want it?
- ◆ Does it fit to your body?
- ◆ Is the spelling correct?
- ◆ Is the design right-side up and facing the right direction?
- ◆ Have you checked it in the mirror? The design should look backward. If it is not, your tattoo will be tattooed backward.

It is really important to take the right steps to be sure that you have the stencil placed perfectly. Remember, this tattoo will be with you forever so placement is key.

> **Tat-tale**
>
> There once was a tattoo patron who wanted to get a Superman logo in the center of his chest. At the tattoo shop, the stencil was placed upon the patron's chest. When the patron looked in the mirror, sure enough, he saw a perfect Superman logo. Unfortunately, he and the tattooist didn't realize that the letters read backward in the mirror, leaving the patron with a permanent, backward Superman logo tattoo.

Drawing It On

Some tattooists prefer to draw on the design with a nontoxic marker such as a Sharpie. Often the artist will start with a light color like yellow and build the drawing up, using a darker color for each layer. This is highly effective for having a design fit well to the shape of your body. Some designs are so simple, like a lady-bug, that it's just more efficient. Script lettering is often drawn on. Rosary beads are much easier to draw on than to stencil well.

For large tattoos, many tattooists will stencil the main subject and then draw on the background. Or for designs with serpentine bodies such as dragons, the artist may stencil the head and feet, and then draw on the body.

Again, every artist has a way of doing things. It's important to be patient, pay attention, and allow the artist to do what she needs to do in order for her to produce the best possible tattoo.

A Few Positions

It is very important for everyone to be comfortable. You need to be comfortable in order to sit still—you will be in enough pain without having to worry about muscle cramps from a weird position. And the artist needs to be comfortable—you don't want him to have a slip of the hand.

Most tattoos are done with you sitting up in a chair with the use of an armrest. That covers forearms, elbows, and upper arms.

For tattoos that fall on the rest of the body, many tattooists will use either a barber's chair that can angle back so you can lie down, or they will use my personal favorite, a massage table. It is much easier to lay people down on a massage table. The tables are reasonably comfortable, and the tattooist can reach any part of the body.

Tattooing Process

For most tattoos, there is a set process artists follow to ensure a quality tattoo. The first step is the outline, next the shading and color, followed by possible retouching or tightening to make sure the tattoo looks amazing. Some tattoos call for a different strategy such as portraits or realistic tattoos. During a portrait, the initial outline may only consist of a few important features such as the eyes or nose. This also may be done using *blood lining*, when the tattooist uses water to tattoo a line. A portrait is mostly shading, so what little lines are made are usually put in the tattoo later.

def•i•ni•tion

Blood lining is when an artist uses water instead of ink to tattoo a line. This is to create a marker on the skin for use later in the tattoo in case the stencil has wiped away.

Outlining

Usually the first step in every tattoo, outlining is the framework of the tattoo. The outline will guide where the shading will be placed. It is important to be still so as not to have a squiggly outline. Most shading can fix a little squiggle, but not all. Outlining is done with a round needle for a consistent line. Rounded needles can also be used to fill in some of the tattoo as well. They are good for the little nooks and crannies such as the tips of a tribal or any little corner.

For larger tattoos, the entire session will be dedicated to just the outline—sometimes using as many as three different needle sizes to have line variation.

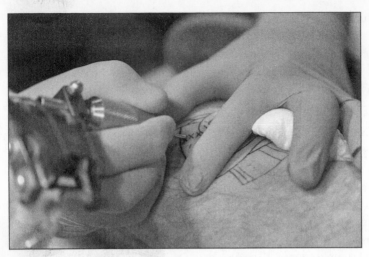

Outlining the tattoo.

Shading

After the outline is complete, it is time to tattoo all the black shading. Black shading is very important as far as making the color in a tattoo appear very bright and intense; this is due to the contrast. The darkness will push the color forward, making it appear much stronger than if the color was on its own. Without black shading, the tattoo will appear slightly faded, especially as the years go by and the tattoo ages.

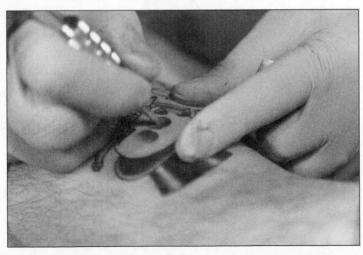

Shading the tattoo.

The same is apparent with black and gray tattoos. Without the dark of the black, the tattoo will appear faded, almost ghostlike. If that is what you are into, then that is perfectly acceptable. It may be that the customer doesn't want the tattoo to stand out but be subtle. In order to have the best tattoo possible, one that will look great for years to come, black is needed.

Once the black is done, it is time for the color. The color is usually done from dark to light. Dark colors are variants of the cool colors such as greens, blues, and purples, while lighter colors are the warm colors such as red, yellow, and orange. Colors that are more pastel, containing more white, will be tattooed after the stronger, more pure colors are applied. This is because the dark colors can get into the already-tattooed lighter colors, affecting the lighter colors. A dark blue can turn a yellow slightly green, for example. White highlights are generally done last, as white pigment can be contaminated the most easily.

Tightening It Up

After the tattoo is finished, the artist will often give it a close examination. This is to check for *holidays*, which are blank spots in the tattoo.

The tattooist will tattoo all the little spots that may have been overlooked. This will yield a more solid tattoo.

def•i•ni•tion

Holidays are little spots of the tattoo that haven't been fully tattooed. When the tattoo is healed, those little spots of bare skin that pop through the tattoo are called holidays.

Some tattooists tighten up tattoos periodically throughout the tattoo. They will shade and color a section of the tattoo then clean it off with soap or water to see the tattooed skin. Then they will tighten up the finished section and move on to the next section.

Touching up the tattoo.

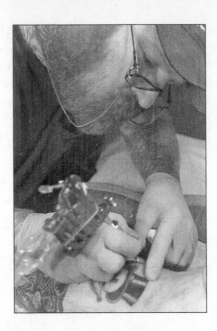

More Than a Feeling: The First Zap

Your design is perfect, the stencil is just right, and the artist has you where you need to be. You are ready for the first zap from the needle, the initial poke you have been wondering about. You will soon see what the hype is all about. Now what do you do as your artist comes at you with that buzzing machine?

Don't jump! Many tattooists give first-timers a quick zap to relieve some of the anxiety that has been building. The first zap is over in less than a second, and you will realize how little a tattoo actually hurts—or how much it really hurts, depending on location. There are a few things you will need to remember to get through the experience with the least amount of hassle.

Relax and Meditate

It is far easier for you and your tattooist to get through the experience if you are relaxed. It is far better to keep your muscles relaxed. Tensing up can lead to your having the shakes, which makes straight lines nearly impossible.

Remember to breathe while you are being tattooed. Many people think it is better to hold their breath while they are getting tattooed. This is not true unless you are getting your stomach or chest tattooed, where the movement of heavy breathing makes tattooing difficult. If you don't breathe, you will pass out.

Try to keep from breathing all over your tattooist. It is very uncomfortable to be breathed on by a stranger. Tattooing can become quite intimate, so be aware of the direction you are exhaling.

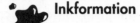 **Inkformation**

An easy, regular breathing pattern will relax you and make it easier for you to deal with getting tattooed.

If you find the feeling uncomfortable, try to meditate or put yourself somewhere else. Daydreaming can help to distract you from the feeling of getting tattooed.

Many people find talking to the artist a good way to distract themselves from the tattoo. The only downside to this is that you don't want to distract your tattooist, because he needs to concentrate.

Many first-timers will bring a friend for support. Clients always say that talking about anything will take their mind away from the tattoo and make the time go by faster. But again, you run the risk of distracting your tattooist.

Sit Still

It is very important that you keep still. One little shake and the whole tattoo can be messed up. Just relax and don't move unless told to. It's best to relax and allow the tattoo to happen. Fighting it only makes it hurt more.

Speak only with your mouth, not with your hands. Any little movement from one part of your body will affect your whole body. This is one of the most common causes of messed up tattoos.

You should have already turned off your cell phone, but if you forgot to, don't jump for it when it rings. Ask the artist if you can answer your phone, or better yet, turn it off.

Passing Out

Passing out happens to many first-timers. It is completely common and a natural thing to do. If you prepare yourself well by eating before you get tattooed, as well as breathing and relaxing during the tattoo, you should be okay. Some people are just prone to passing out. If you are one of those people, tell your artist. She will understand and can keep you from completely blacking out by stopping the tattoo while someone in the shop gets you some water. It takes about ten minutes of you relaxing in the chair for the feeling to pass.

Signs of Passing Out

It is easy to tell if you are going to pass out. The signs are there, every time. Most people try to tough it out, thinking it will pass. It will pass, but after you have hit the floor and have possibly puked all over the place. The signs of passing out include the following:

◆ Light-headedness

◆ Cold sweats

◆ Face turning pale green

If you don't tell the tattooist to stop or hint at how you feel, the tattooist may not notice and you will pass out.

Don't be afraid to tell the tattooist you feel you are going to pass out. Otherwise you might collapse and hurt yourself—or worse, vomit on your tattooist.

If you feel you have to vomit, aim for the garbage can, which should be near you. It's easier to change a garbage bag than to mop a floor or tattoo someone covered in vomit.

What to Do if You Pass Out

If you do pass out, don't worry. People pass out all the time. You will wake up not knowing what planet you are on for only a few seconds. Pretty soon you'll be conscious, feeling a little silly for passing out. Be sure to …

♦ Drink some water.

♦ Stay where you are; if you get up, you might collapse and hit your head on something.

♦ Breathe in through your nose, out through your mouth.

♦ Relax and don't worry about it.

♦ Continue the tattoo when you have completely recovered.

If you pass out, you will only pass out one time, usually toward the beginning of the tattoo. On very rare occasions people have gone down twice, but they hadn't eaten and had taken some kind of pills and alcohol. Most people feel much better after passing out and are ready to go in five to ten minutes. Again, don't be afraid to take a few minutes to fully recover. You will feel much better.

Taking Breaks

During larger tattoos, it is normal to take a break or two. Smaller tattoos are done so quickly, there won't be enough time for a break. However, if you feel you need to rest for a moment, don't be afraid to ask for a break. Tattooists who are smokers will often take cigarette breaks. Often you may need to use the bathroom or get something to drink.

Don't be afraid to ask for a break if you have been sitting for over an hour. Many artists will take a break after the outline or after all the black is done. This enables you to

Inkformation

The longer the break you take, the more it hurts when you start again because you have to get used to the feeling again. This time, however, you are getting tattooed on already-tattooed, swollen skin.

stretch, take a look in the mirror, smoke a cigarette, or whatever you can do in five minutes. While you do whatever you do, the tattooist can prepare for the next part of the tattoo or just go chat with the other tattooists.

Bandages

Now you have survived your first tattoo. It feels good to be done. The tattooist will have you look at the tattoo in the mirror so you can see it for the first time. This is usually the best part of the tattoo because you can see the end results of all that went into this experience.

Take a look at your new tattoo in the mirror before the tattooist puts a bandage on it.

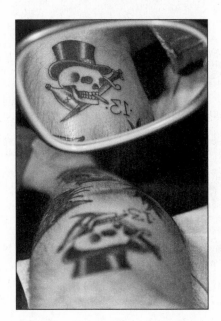

Now the tattooist will clean the tattoo with soap. He will get off all of the excess ink and blood. A tattoo is an open wound, so it is important that it is properly cleaned before being bandaged. Also the tattooed area will be too sensitive hours later to try to scrub off any unwashed ink stains from your skin.

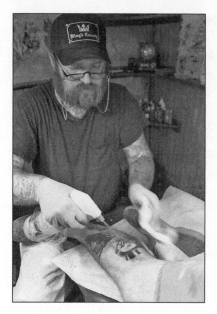

Before wrapping the tattoo, Chops cleans it with green soap.

A thin layer of ointment will be applied to your tattoo to keep the bandage from sticking to the tattoo. Bandages are important because they keep dirt and bacteria from getting on the fresh tattoo. Also, bandages keep your blood, which will be slowly seeping out of the tattoo, from getting all over your clothes and whatever else you come into contact with.

There are a few different types of bandage options:

- **Plastic wrap.** Some tattooists use plastic wrap because it sticks well to your skin and enables you and your friends to see the fresh tattoo. Plastic wrap stays put better than bandages on moving parts of the body such as a shoulder or knee.

- **Absorbent bandage.** Sometimes absorbent bandages such as gauze pads are used because they absorb the blood well and are comfortable against the skin.

- **Paper towels.** A simple paper towel can also be used to cover a tattoo. It is quick and easy, but may stick to the tattoo.

Each form of bandage is held on with bandage tape or masking tape. All these devices work well to protect a new tattoo from the environment.

Bandaging the tattoo.

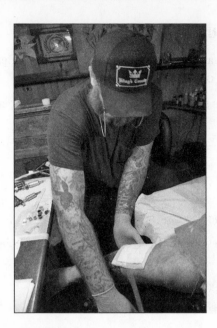

Payment and Tipping

Your fresh tattoo is all done. You have joined the "club" and are ready to show off your new acquisition. Time to pay. Some tattoo shops have you pay before the tattoo. This is a protection for them just in case a credit card doesn't work or something else goes wrong. Most shops will take credit and debit cards, but some are cash only. In some shops the tattooist will accept the payment, while in others the floor person or manager will take care of it.

If you are really pleased with the tattoo, it is polite to tip the tattooist. The tip is a sign of your gratitude for the work you just received. Usually about 10 percent of the total is more than enough. Many shops have signs on the wall to remind customers about tipping. However, it is not necessary to tip the tattooist. Only tip if you are really happy with the tattoo and you have extra to give. Tattoos are not cheap, and tattooists understand that we all have bills to pay.

The Least You Need to Know

- ◆ Prepare yourself both physically and mentally before the tattoo.

- ◆ Your skin must be shaved and disinfected first to ensure a clean tattoo.

- ◆ Always double-check the spelling of your tattoo.

- ◆ Relax, remain still, and stay in position to avoid mistakes.

- ◆ Passing out is not uncommon for first-timers—you should be fine in five to ten minutes.

- ◆ There are a few different products used to bandage a tattoo such as plastic wrap, gauze pads, or just a paper towel.

Chapter 13

Now You Are Tattooed

In This Chapter

- ◆ Taking care of the fresh tattoo
- ◆ Keeping the tattoo looking good
- ◆ Next tattoo
- ◆ Covering the old tattoos
- ◆ Laser removal

It feels good to get out of the chair or off the massage table after the tattooist says that you are finished. There is nothing like the feeling of being done with getting a tattoo. Now you can show all your friends and maybe your parents. You are now "one of those people" who has a tattoo and there is no going back.

The process isn't over yet, though. Now you need to care for the tattoo. As you will see, there are a few steps to the aftercare that you will need to follow. There are also a few steps to ensure that your tattoo will look good for years to come.

Usually after the first tattoo, the next idea will start floating around in your thoughts … so you may need to make another trip to the tattoo shop. Tattoos are addictive. In this chapter we will go over what you need to do to take care of your tattoo and the different methods of changing your tattoo or having it removed.

Aftercare

The tattoo is done and the job of the tattooist is complete. Now it is your turn to take care of the tattoo. It is extremely important that you take good care of a healing tattoo. How you care for the tattoo will affect how the tattoo looks for the rest of your life. Proper care of a tattoo will ensure that the tattoo has bright colors and dark blacks.

Every tattoo shop will tell you a different way to take care of a tattoo. Each method is basically the same. Some people disagree on what to use, what not to use, or what is best to put on the tattoo. What matters is that the tattoo heals up without any reactions. Let's take a look at the basic method of taking care of a fresh tattoo.

What to Do

Once completed, the tattooist will place a bandage over the tattoo. This is to protect it from dirt and other foreign objects. It also keeps your clothes or anything else from rubbing against your sensitive tattoo. You will want to keep the bandage on for at least two hours. Many tattooists suggest that you keep the bandage on overnight so the tattoo won't stick to your sheets or pajamas. Some of the ink will seep out of your skin during the first 12 hours and stain whatever you are wearing or sleeping on.

If you shower before going to bed, wash the tattoo and then cautiously tape a piece of plastic wrap over the tattoo. Plastic wrap makes a great protective cover for tattoos. Tattoos on some parts of the body, such as the chest, can be hard to keep bandages on, as they will fall off with your body movements. You can either retape the bandage on or just take it off and go to the next step.

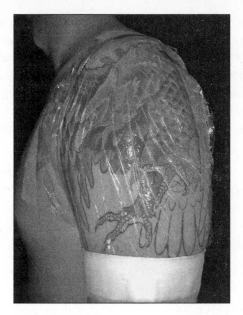

Plastic wrap makes a great bandage and is good for rewrapping a fresh tattoo to keep the tattoo from becoming more irritated.

After the bandage has come off, you will need to clean your tattoo. There will be some tattoo color slime that has oozed out of your skin along with a little blood. This is normal. Wash the tattoo gently with soap and water. Most of the time it is just easier to take a shower. Many tattoos are on body parts that make washing in a sink very awkward.

There is a great technique that can really help the healing of your tattoo. While you are washing your tattoo, you will notice that it feels like a sunburn and is very sensitive to warm water. Let the warm water run over your fresh tattoo until the tattoo gets used to the temperature of the water. Once the water doesn't burn, turn up the temperature just a little so it irritates the tattoo again. Repeat this until the temperature of the water is just a little hotter than what you would consider a hot shower. This process will open the pores in the skin of your tattoo and wash out all of the dirt and excess ink. It will also get rid of a lot of the irritation your skin will have from getting tattooed. You may find that doing this once after you get tattooed will help your tattoo heal faster and better.

After you wash your tattoo for the first time, don't moisturize it with anything. Let it dry. Then you may want to cover the tattoo with a piece of plastic wrap. It isn't necessary to do so, but it will keep the tattoo from getting irritated by anything that could rub up against it like your clothes or a family pet. You will want to change the plastic wrap once or twice throughout the day. That is up to your discretion. Wrap your tattoo with plastic wrap before going to bed on the next night. It will again keep the tattoo from sticking to your sheets.

> **Tat-tale**
>
> On the following night, after getting a fresh tattoo on his forearm, a young man went to bed with his young wife nestled over his tattooed arm so he could hold her. The next morning they awoke to find the tattoo stuck to the side of the young beautiful wife's face. After removing the arm from the face, the wife was left with a full color print of the tattoo stretched across the side of her face. Don't worry, it washed off in the shower.

On the following night, a full 24 hours after you have been tattooed, you will want to wash the tattoo again, just with soap and warm water. After the tattoo has dried, you must moisturize the tattoo with one of the following products before rewrapping it with plastic wrap:

- ◆ A&D Ointment
- ◆ Bacitracin (Neosporin will work, but due to the many chemicals in it, it may not react well)
- ◆ Tattoo Goo or other tattoo-company treatments (these are usually sold in tattoo shops and are great for tattoos but will cost at least double what it costs to buy Bacitracin)
- ◆ Bepanthen (found in Europe and works really well)
- ◆ Basic perfume-free skin moisturizer (but nothing with aloe or any chemical additives) and topical vitamins (such as vitamin E or D)

The point of moisturizing the tattoo is to keep it from drying out, which would make it hard for your skin to heal. You just want to moisturize the tattoo as if you were moisturizing your hands.

Don't leave globs of moisturizer on your fingers; rub it in so there is no excess. Too much ointment on your new tattoo will draw the ink out of your skin and the tattoo won't heal as bright or as dark as it should. Also, after the excess ointment draws the ink out of your skin, it will dry into a thick scab. If the thick scab is pulled off prematurely, it will leave a blank spot in your tattoo, which will then need a touch-up. So remember to wipe off the excess ointment, or it will ruin your tattoo.

Flash Tip

If you accidentally put too much ointment on and you see ink coming out of your skin, wash it off with soap and warm water before it dries. Washing the ink off will keep the ink from causing a scab.

You will need to moisturize your tattoo with one of the various products three or four times a day for four or five days. The number of times a day depends on you. If the tattoo feels dry, then moisturize it. Usually the various products like A&D ointment are used until the scabs have flaked off. After that, just use a regular skin moisturizer for at least a week.

Due to many people having an allergic reaction to petroleum-based products such as A&D ointment, Bacitracin, and the various tattoo-company products (read the labels for the ingredients) many tattooists will suggest using a basic skin moisturizer that doesn't have any perfume or aloe, which is a natural astringent, throughout the whole process. All that other stuff works well, but all you really need is to use basic moisturizer for two or three weeks.

Inkformation

Petroleum-based products or ointments that have an oily consistency can feel uncomfortable on your skin when the weather is humid.

The Do Nots

Your tattoo will scab. Usually it will peel like a sunburn but sometimes it won't peel at all. Do not pick the scabs. Your skin is still healing beneath the scabs. If you pick the scabs off, you can cause scarring, and as we saw before, you can pick holes and ruin your tattoo.

Do not go swimming. If your tattoo becomes too moist, from too much ointment or being submerged in water for too long, ink will come out of your skin. Chlorinated water found in pools will react badly with your tattoo. It can cause irritation and then create excess scabbing.

Do not get direct sunlight on your tattoo. As we have seen, the sun will mess up your tattoo. If you work outdoors, wear something that will cover your new tattoo. If the tattoo is on an arm, you can cut the end off of a clean sock and slide that over your tattoo. The beach is a no-no, as there isn't usually any cover from the sun and you can't go swimming with the new tattoo anyway. To be safe, you will want to keep a new tattoo out of the sun for three weeks to a month, and you will want to put an SPF 45 sunblock on it. It is usually a better idea to get tattooed in the fall or winter so you don't have to worry about a missed opportunity to go to the beach.

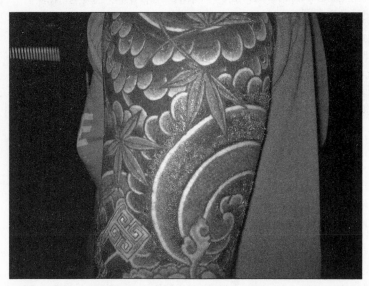

Your tattoo may peel like a sunburn.

Do not scratch your tattoo. As the tattoo is healing, it will begin to itch. If you scratch the tattoo while it is healing, you could rip a scab off prematurely and cause a holiday in the tattoo. You could just tear the skin, as it is very thin and more delicate than normal while it is healing. You can slap the tattoo, which will cause some relief. The best way to avoid a very itchy tattoo is to moisturize it properly throughout the healing process.

Larger tattoos that take up a lot of skin and are near a joint will take longer to heal if the joint gets too much movement while the tattoo is trying to heal. You will feel the irritation. It is best to avoid working out for a few days. If you are in some kind of self-defense class like karate, kung fu, or kickboxing, you may want to avoid getting hit near the area of the tattoo. You also may want to take it easy on the calisthenics. Many construction workers and mechanics will get tattooed on a Friday evening so they have the whole weekend to heal. It's best to take it easy for a few a days to let your tattoo heal properly.

Healing Time

All tattoos heal at different rates. Tattoos on parts of the body that have a lot of movement like the wrist or elbow may take longer to heal. Your health will determine the healing time as well. Some tattooists have a heavier hand, which means they use more pressure and run their machines harder so their tattoos can sometimes take longer to heal, especially if the tattoos are not properly taken care of.

Usually after two or three days, the tattoo will begin to scab or peel. It takes anywhere from a few days to a week for this to finish. A scab can be stubborn and stay on for over three weeks, but that is usually in an area that takes longer to heal.

After the scabs have flaked away, your skin will appear shiny. This is because it is still healing. The new skin of the tattoo will feel softer, thinner, and more delicate during this time. It will be that way for about a month. If you need to have a touch-up or want to add on to your tattoo or change something in the design, you will have to wait well over a month before the skin is ready to be tattooed again. When the tattoo looks like it is 100 percent part of your skin, then you can have it worked on again. If you don't wait, you could cause scarring, and the new ink may not stay in. If that happens, the tattoo will take even longer to heal, and you will have to get the new tattoo work done again, which would then take much longer than simply waiting those initial few weeks.

Skin and Body Reactions

You will notice that your body will react to getting tattooed. As we know, everyone reacts differently, but here are a few basic reactions that you may or may not notice. The area under and around the tattoo will bruise, so you will see a slight brown tinting under and around your tattoo while it is healing. Sometimes the bruise will go beyond the tattooed area like a halo. The area that has been tattooed will swell and be sore as if something hit you forcefully. If you have been tattooed on or near a joint, that joint may become sore when you move it.

Again, the tattooed skin will feel like a sunburn, and will be very sensitive to the touch. Your skin will feel very taut and may not allow you to stretch; it may feel like your skin will tear. You also may have a reaction to the ink, which we went over in Chapter 4. A bad reaction is very rare so you don't need to worry about that too much. If you have a bad reaction, get in touch with your tattooist so they can tell you how to take care of it or go see your doctor.

Getting large amounts of skin tattooed at once can lower your immune system, which can lead to you coming down with a cold or flu. This usually only happens if you get over eight hours of work done at once. Some people travel very far to get tattooed by a specific person. They will often get tattooed for two days in a row, for many hours at a time. This can really lower your immune system. If you are going to do this, remember to eat healthfully and bring lots of vitamins.

The Effects of the Sun

The sun's ultraviolet rays will age your tattoo as well as give you skin cancer if you aren't careful. The UV rays are very harmful to a new tattoo. The skin of a new tattoo is trying to heal and get used to all the ink. It doesn't have all of its usual defenses to protect you from the sun.

If you expose your tattoo to the sun, it will heal poorly. First the skin will burn, then the tattoo will start to look pale, and a white coat of dead skin will form. The tattoo will feel thick and raised as the color seems to recede and fade. The tattoo will then scab thickly and crack, and take much longer to heal. Your tattoo will lose a lot of its color and contrast, and most likely need to be done over. In other words, you will want to keep your tattoo out of the sun. It's not a pretty sight.

Tattoos Age in the Sun

You have seen that the sun will ruin your tattoo. Have you ever noticed how old signs left in the sun are faded as if they have been bleached? Ultraviolet rays fade pigment whether it's on a piece of wood or in your skin. Have you ever noticed that art museums with paintings have no open windows where the sun can directly shine in? The sun would destroy millions of dollars' worth of artwork. You won't want your artwork destroyed, either, so use a good, strong sunblock when going out in the sun.

Tanning Beds

If you go to tanning salons often, you might as well skip getting any form of serious tattooing. You will ruin the tattoo quickly. Tanning beds are as unhealthy as smoking and fast food, but it is your life. If you don't mind having a faded tattoo or are willing to have it done over every five years to keep it looking decent, go for it. You can always put some sunblock on the tattoo before you tan.

Keeping Your Tattoo Healthy

Keeping your tattoo healthy is easy. If you are a person who generally takes good care of your skin, you won't have any problems taking care of your tattoo. If you don't pay much attention to your skin's health, that's okay, but just pay attention to the tattoo. Keep your tattoo moist by rubbing moisturizer on it daily. If you are in a dry climate or are prone to dry skin, you will want to moisturize at least twice a day. Use a very strong sunblock, such as SPF 45 or stronger, when you are in the sun. Eat healthfully, too. The healthier you are, the healthier your tattoos will be.

Making the Next Appointment

When you are getting large tattoos, you will need a few appointments. Tattooists who are good at planning ahead will set you up with as many appointments as they feel they will need to finish the tattoo. This is good for you. Some tattooists are very booked up with appointments, and you may have to wait weeks, months, or even a year until your next appointment. If you can get the appointments in advance, you won't have to wait and you can complete your tattoo as quickly as possible.

You may need to wait until the tattoo is healed before continuing, which may take more than a month. Many people will just work on different sections of the tattoo so that you can get tattooed weekly. Usually one week for an outline to heal is long enough to continue with the shading.

Some customers know that they will want to get another tattoo right after they get their first one. If this happens to you, you can make your next appointment before you walk out the door. Many tattooists take this as a compliment, showing that you particularly liked their work.

Spreading the Word

If you have followed the guidance of this book and really made the right choices, chances are you should be pretty happy with your new tattoo. Now you can help guide people who don't know where to go for a tattoo. Don't be afraid to show your tattoo in public. Wear clothing that will show off your new tattoo if you can. You will meet many other tattoo enthusiasts and you can share your tattoo experiences with each other.

Remember to grab some business cards from your tattooist or tattoo shop. If you keep them in your wallet or in your purse, you can hand them out when someone asks you about your tattoos. Many shops have free stickers, too. Stick them around town or on your car. Give them to friends. Buy one of your tattoo shop's t-shirts or sweat shirts—these are shirts not many people will have, so you will have something fairly original to wear in public.

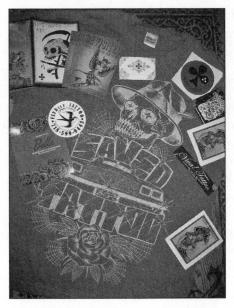

Here are a few examples of items you can pick up from a tattoo shop to help support them.

The Internet is a great place to brag about your tattoo. You can put a photo of your tattoo on MySpace or another social website. There are hundreds of tattoo chat rooms you can visit if you want to share your experience. You may want to talk about your tattoo on your blog, as getting it was a new experience that has physically changed you. Your tattooist will appreciate your enthusiasm and definitely appreciate all the new business you bring him.

Touch-Ups

Sometimes things happen and a tattoo needs a touch-up. It's a normal part of tattooing that even the most experienced tattooist will need to do. As we have seen, your tattoo must be fully healed in order for it to be tattooed again. Usually a month will do if you take really good care of it, but sometimes it is a few weeks longer.

Touch-ups are usually free as long as the tattoo looks like you have been taking care of it. If you let it roast in the sun, let it dry out, pick the scabs, or put way too much ointment on it, a tattooist will be able to tell. She may tell you that you need to pay to have it fixed, as it is not her fault the tattoo was not taken care of.

It is the responsibility of the tattooist who did the tattoo to do the touch-up, not the shop's responsibility. If you go to someone else, he will charge you or he may not do it—some tattooists consider it taboo for a tattooist to work on someone else's tattoo. Many times a shop will do the touch-up if the tattooist is out of town. Or they may make an appointment with the tattooist for you to have it touched up. If you know you are going to get another tattoo by the same tattooist, you may want to wait for a touch-up until then. It is easier to get two birds with one stone. Tattooists and tattoo shops usually care about their reputation and will want the tattoo to be as perfect as possible.

Getting Rid of That Old Tattoo

Many people find that they want to get rid of their old tattoos. There are many reasons for wanting to get rid of old designs. Lots of people make immature decisions when they are young and find the tattoo embarrassing when they get older. A weed leaf may be cool when you are 18 but hard to show your future mother-in-law. Having an ex-lover's name can really make for an interesting time with your new significant other.

Some people get very poorly done tattoos that look like they were done in jail by a hack—or were actually done in jail by a hack. These tattoos are often embarrassing and look horrible, and they will need changing. Or the person may feel the style is outdated or he just doesn't like the style he chose anymore, and so he wants to have a new style placed over the old one. Smaller tattoos often end up looking too small, so they can either be added onto or covered with something larger that fits the body much better. Let's look at the different options to changing old and unwanted tattoos.

Covering It Up

Getting an old tattoo covered up with a new one is becoming more and more popular. Every tattooist has to learn how to do cover ups. Doing a good cover up is not easy. On many cover-ups you can still see a little hint of the old tattoo behind the new one. That is normal. Some cover-ups are over very dark or heavily scarred tattoos. There is nothing that can be done for the texture of the scarring in the old tattoo but the old tattoo design can be made illegible.

A cover-up is an entirely different tattoo than a tattoo on blank skin. Some concepts work in covering up tattoos, but most concepts don't work when covering tattoos. There are a few important things you should know if you want to get a good cover-up so that the new tattoo looks like a good tattoo and not like a cover-up.

- The new tattoo design must be at least three or four times the size of your old tattoo.

- The new tattoo will need to use plenty of black shading, especially if the old tattoo is really dark.

- The new tattoo design must be a solid design with lots of coverage. You won't be able to have negative spaces in the tattoo, so typical tribal designs will not work.

- Flash designs usually don't work well for larger cover-ups, but there are a few exceptions. Usually a design will have to be custom-drawn to ensure the old tattoo is covered up completely.

- Warm colors like red, yellow, and orange don't work well for covering tattoos. Cool colors like blue, green, and purple are needed to cover old tattoos.

- It may take a second or third layer of tattooing to completely cover your old tattoo if it is really dark. Therefore, you need to have patience when getting this done.

Choosing an idea for your cover-up design can be difficult. Not all ideas will work due to all the limitations of getting a cover-up.

Many times a cover-up will simply camouflage the old tattoo. This is easier to do with tattoos that have a lot of detail. Any animal or mythological beast that has scales or feathers is a good choice for a cover-up. Asian-style dragons, koi fish, or any kind of fish that can be darkly shaded will work well. Also, birds such as ravens or eagles will make for good cover-ups. As we saw before, biomechanical tattoos can have a lot of detail and are good for cover-ups.

Flash Tip

One or two sessions of laser removal can lighten up your old tattoo enough to allow for a wider array of design options for a cover-up.

A design that has a dark robe like a Grimm Reaper will be able to cover most other designs. You could replace the Grimm Reaper with a woman in a cloak, and use her hair to help with the cover-up. Seventeenth-century French ornamental design can work well if it is put together correctly. Dark floral designs that have a lot of dark leaves are good, and may work if you need a name in a banner covered. Most of the time you will need to cover the entire tattoo and not just the name.

For background on cover-ups, black atmospheric shading works well. An example of this can be seen in classical Chinese brush painting. There are no rigid lines or rules of how to put it together like in traditional Japanese backgrounds. This gives the tattooist the freedom to place the shading where she needs to, to further cover the old tattoo. It is also faster to accomplish and will hurt less in the end.

When getting a cover-up, you will need a consultation. The tattooist will usually make a tracing of the area and the old tattoo so that he will know what it looks like while he draws the new design to cover the old one. Many tattooists will draw on you to get a feel for what needs to be done, and then take a digital picture of that for later reference. Some cover-ups need to be drawn on completely without the use of a stencil. This works well because the design will fit to the body well and you will be able to see how it is done. Every tattooist has his own way of solving cover-ups.

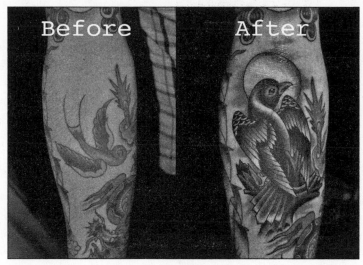

An example of an old, unwanted tattoo and then the tattoo that covered it up.

Not all cover-ups need to be so elaborate. Older tattoos that have faded to almost nothing after years in the sun or tattoos that have had a turn under the laser machine are easier to cover. Still, you will want to research well who does your cover-up. Cover-up tattoos can be very expensive due to the amount of work and concentration needed to get them done and done well.

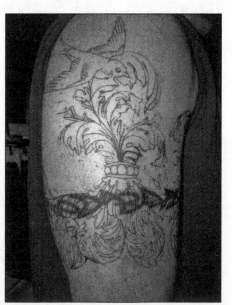

An example of a stencil over an old tattoo that is about to be covered.

Lasering It Off

The best way to get rid of your old tattoo is to have it removed by laser. Laser removal works by a quick pulse of highly concentrated light that breaks up the tattoo pigment in your skin. The smaller particles of pigment are then taken away by your immune system.

Laser removal is a great way to get rid of a tattoo, but it can leave scarring or a discoloration of your skin. Also, the tattoo may never totally disappear. You may be left with a few light spots of tattoo. Laser treatment is also very painful. It will hurt about four times more than getting the tattoo in the first place. However, the treatment is fast and may only take a few minutes. After the treatment is done, the treated skin will be sore and may scab. You will have to wait for the skin to heal before going back for another treatment.

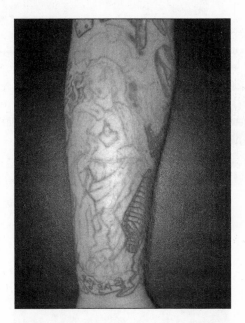

Laser treatment will take a few sessions to be completed. This tattoo has had two sessions.

Tattoos that were done by the inexperienced may take longer to laser. If the tattoo was done poorly, the ink might be on different layers of the dermis, whereas an experienced professional will have the ink inserted on just about the same level. Blue and black ink are the easiest to remove. Black will absorb all of the different kinds of intense light used to remove tattoos, so the black ink particles will break up more easily. Yellows and greens are harder to break up and may take more treatments.

Laser removal is not cheap. It takes many sessions, which can cost $250 and up, per session, depending on the size of the tattoo. Health insurance usually won't cover the cost, either, as it is a cosmetic surgery. If you want to get laser removal, do some research when looking for a place to have it done. Some places will have better results than others and be more efficient.

Inkformation

There are other products out there that say they remove tattoos. If you want to try them, do some research first. Many postings on the Internet say that the products only lightened the tattoos just enough to help with a cover-up, but it took many months. Other postings say that nothing happened at all and the companies wouldn't return phone calls. Many tattooists swear by laser removal and have had it done themselves.

The Least You Need to Know

◆ You will want to keep your tattoo moisturized during the healing process.

◆ It can take up to two weeks for your tattoo to heal, but take over a month for your tattoo to completely heal in order to rework the area.

◆ Use SPF 45 or higher on your tattoo when you go out in the sun.

◆ To get your old tattoo covered with a new one, the new design must be three or four times the size of the older tattoo.

◆ Laser surgery is the best way to remove a tattoo to date, but it is very painful and can be quite expensive.

Glossary

A&D ointment A petroleum-based product that contains vitamins A and D and can be used to heal a tattoo as well as diaper rash.

AIDS Acquired Immunodeficiency Syndrome is caused by the retrovirus HIV because your body's immune system cannot defend itself against infection.

armature bar The long rectangular piece of metal on a tattoo machine that is pulled up and down by the turning on and off of an electromagnetic coil. The armature bar also holds the eye-loop end of the needle bar.

asymmetrical A term used to describe a design that is not identical on both sides or that is not symmetrical.

autoclave A hospital-grade sterilizer that uses steam and pressure to sterilize equipment.

bacitracin A petroleum-based antibiotic topical cream that can be used to heal your tattoo.

Bepanthen An antiseptic cream that can be used to heal your tattoo.

bilirubin A yellow breakdown product of red blood cells that can be seen in the yellowing of a bruise, jaundice, and the brownish-yellow color of feces.

biomechanical   An artistic style that involves the combination of organic form and industrial form, which can be seen in the artwork of H. R. Giger.

blackletter   A form of writing that was created around 1150 C.E. so that books could be produced by hand at a faster rate.

bloodline   When the tattooist makes a line in the skin with water so he will have a guide for the shading later in the tattoo process.

blow-out   A shadow on the line of the tattoo that occurs when the tattoo liner needle goes into the skin in the wrong direction. It is a common occurrence in tattooing.

body suit   A tattoo or a collection of tattoos that cover the torso or an entire body. Body suits are usually associated with Japanese style tattooing.

Carolingian Minuscule   A form of handwriting that was developed around 800 C.E. for use in manuscripts.

clip cord   The cord that is attached to the back of the tattoo machine to feed the machine electricity.

connective tissue   The tissue in the body that is involved in structure and support.

collagen   The main protein of connective tissue.

coils   The two cylinder-shaped pieces on traditional tattoo machines. They are electromagnets and pull down the armature bar when activated.

consultation   A meeting with the tattooist to plan out your tattoo and make a deposit for an appointment.

cover-up   When a new tattoo is tattooed over an old tattoo.

cross-contamination   The transference of a matter from one surface to the other, such as blood from a tattoo transferred from the skin to a counter top via a latex glove.

dermis   The second layer of skin where the pigment from a tattoo is held in place.

eczema   A broad term for inflammation of the skin, such as a recurring rash.

elastin   An elastic-like protein that enables skin to stretch and contract, yet still resume its original shape.

electromagnet   A type of magnet that creates a magnetic field with the flow of an electrical current.

epidermis   The top layer of skin.

flash   Tattoo designs that are created for multiple uses and are displayed in the tattoo shop in flash racks, on the wall, or in books.

foot pedal   A pedal that is used to turn a tattoo machine on or off.

glucocorticoid hormones   A form of steroid hormone that keeps the skin from producing collagen and elastin, which are key to keeping rapidly growing skin firm.

green soap   A type of soap that is typically used in tattoo shops to clean the skin and the tattoo.

grip   This is the "handle" of the tube. It allows for easier maneuvering of the machine.

hanya mask   A mask used in traditional Japanese Noh Theater. It is characterized by having two pointed horns and sharp teeth much like a western devil. The image is also used to scare off evil spirits by hanging it on a wall in your house or having it tattooed on your body.

helper T cells   A type of white blood cell that activates and directs other cells in the immune system.

Hepatitis   A term used to describe an inflammation of the cells in your liver. It can be brought on by drug and alcohol abuse, the digestion of a poisonous mushroom, cancer, and many other situations. The symptoms of Hepatitis are like the flu. It will also cause jaundice, yellowing of the skin and eyes.

HIV   Human Immunodeficiency Virus is a virus that attacks the helper T cells in your blood and will cause AIDS.

holiday   A spot in a tattoo where the ink has fallen out during the healing process.

hypodermis   The third layer of skin that is mainly for storing fat and holding some proteins. The thickness of the hypodermis depends on the amount of fat stored in the body.

hypertrophic scars   Scars that heal a little puffy. They are raised up but not solid. With hypertrophic scars, the regenerating skin cells grow larger than they should.

irezumi   The Japanese term for tattooing. It translates roughly to placing pigment under the skin to permanently leave a decorative mark.

jaundice   A yellowing of the skin and eyes created by an overabundance of bilirubin in the blood.

keratin   A tough, fibrous, structural protein that can be found in the epidermis.

keyloid   A scar that occurs when the collagen made to repair the abrasion grows out of control. A keyloid scar is firm and rubbery and can grow into a benign tumorous growth.

laser removal   The removal of a tattoo with intense pulses of light. Often much more expensive and much more painful than the original tattoo.

liner needle   The needle used to line a tattoo.

Matacide   A surface cleaner that kills germs and viruses such as *E. coli* or HIV.

magnum shader   The most commonly used needle in shading a tattoo. A magnum shader is a flat shading needle in which the pins are spread apart to make it easier to tattoo.

melanin   A dark pigment made by your skin to protect your skin from the harmful rays of the sun.

melanocyte   The skin cell that resides at the bottom of your epidermis and creates melanin.

muscular hypertrophy   A term used in science for the growth and increase of muscle mass.

needle bar   The long bar that the tattoo needle is soldered to.

needle grouping   A group of pins soldered together to make a larger needle to tattoo with.

Old English   A font that is very popular to have tattooed. Gang members of all kinds will often use it when having words tattooed on them.

one-point tattoo   A tattoo that is usually done in one session and can be seen from one vantage point.

phagocytes   A cell that ingests and destroys foreign matter. In tattooing, these cells engulf the color particle and then hold the color particle in place while your skin heals.

pigment   The colored powder material that is the base of all paints and inks.

pins   The individual sharps that are soldered together to make a tattoo needle.

psoriasis   A disease which affects the skin and joints. It usually causes the skin to become red and scaly.

release form   The form you will fill out that legally states you are allowing the tattooist to tattoo you, and protects the tattooist from lawsuits.

"s" curve   A design concept in which the basic shape of the design or parts of the design are in the shape of an "s."

script   A form of handwriting that is a very popular lettering for tattoos.

shader needle   A needle that is used for shading a tattoo.

sharps container   A container that is used to store used needles until they are properly disposed of.

skin   An organ that is made up of three layers: the epidermis, the dermis, and the hypodermis.

stencil   A copy of your design, which is usually in outline form. Tattooists use stencils to give you a good idea of what the tattoo will look like on your body before you get started.

stencil machine   The machine that makes the stencil through a heat process.

symmetrical   A term used to describe designs that are identical on both sides.

tube   The part that is held by the tattooist in his or her hands. It holds and guides the needle as well as gives the machine something to attach to.

ultrasonic cleaner   A machine that is basically a small tub of water that vibrates all the particles out of the tube.

Flash Designs

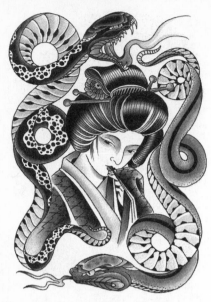

(Courtesy of Alex McWatt, alexmcwatt.com)

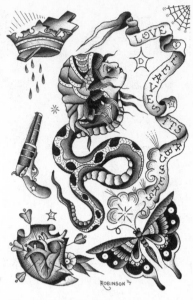

(Courtesy of Bailey Robinson, Hold Fast Tattoo, Brooklyn, NY, www.holdfastbrooklyn.com)

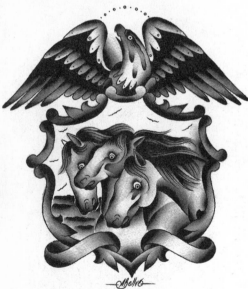

(Courtesy of Aaron Believe, Totem Tattoo Studios, Williamsport, PA)

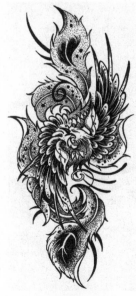

(Courtesy of Miki Foged, Miami Custom Tattoo)

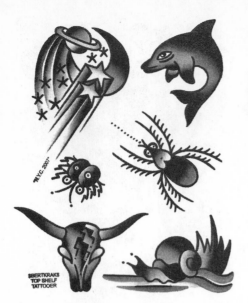

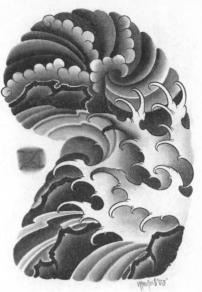

(Courtesy of Bert Krak, Top Shelf Tattooing, Queens, NY, www.bertkrak.com

(Courtesy of Brian Mac, Cobra Custom Tattoo, Plymouth, MA, cobracustomtattoo.com)

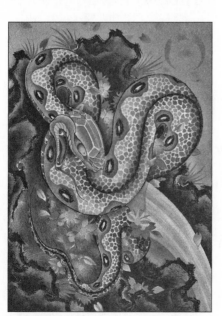

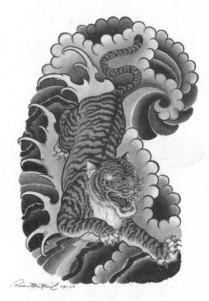

(Courtesy of Brian Mac, Cobra Custom Tattoo, Plymouth, MA, cobracustomtattoo.com)

(Courtesy of Brian Mac, Cobra Custom Tattoo, Plymouth, MA, cobracustomtattoo.com)

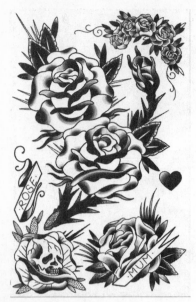

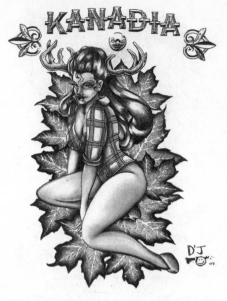

(Courtesy of Ian "Bugsy" Christiansen, Evil from the Needle, London, England, www.myspace.com/ xbugsxstaceyxtattoosx)

(Courtesy of D'Joe, Lark Tattoo, Westbury, NY, www.larktattoo.com)

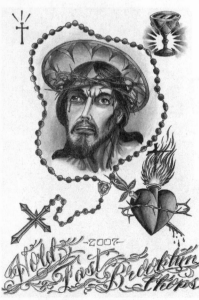

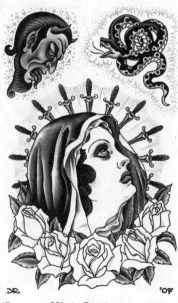

(Courtesy of Katja Ramirez, Houston, Texas, www.kotattoos.com)

(Courtesy of Chops, Hold Fast Tattoo, Brooklyn, NY, www.holdfastbrooklyn.com)

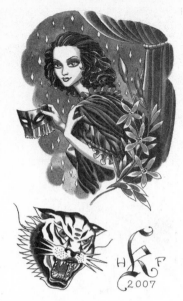

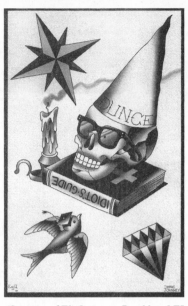

*(Courtesy of Kelly Krantz,
Hold Fast Tattoo, Brooklyn, NY,
www.holdfastbrooklyn.com)*

*(Courtesy of Eli Quinters, Brooklyn, NY,
www.tattoosfortheunloved.com)*

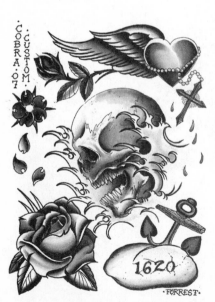

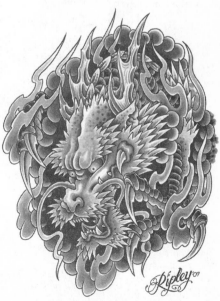

*(Courtesy of Forrest, Cobra Custom Tattoo,
Plymouth, MA, cobracustomtattoo.com)*

*(Courtesy of Judd Ripley, Royal Tattoo,
Helsignør, DK, www.juddripley.com)*

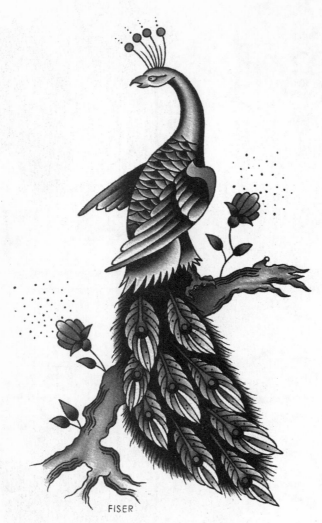

(Courtesy of Barrett Fiser, www.heavysolids.com)

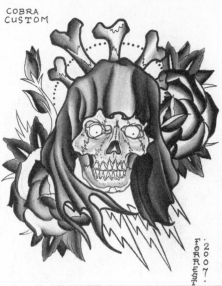

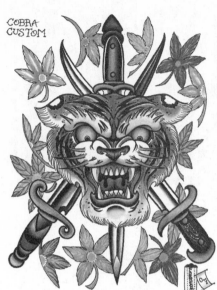

(Courtesy of Forrest, Cobra Custom Tattoo, Plymouth, MA, cobracustomtattoo.com)

(Courtesy of Forrest, Cobra Custom Tattoo, Plymouth, MA, cobracustomtattoo.com)

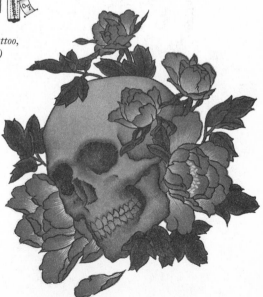

(Courtesy of Brian Mac, Cobra Custom Tattoo, Plymouth, MA, cobracustomtattoo.com)

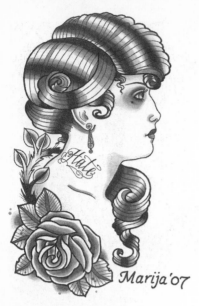

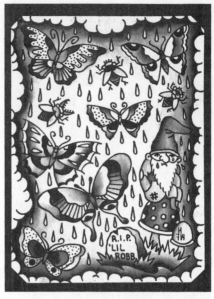

(Courtesy of Marija Asanovski, Royal Tattoo, Helsignør, DK, www.royaltattoo.com)

(Courtesy of Hillary Fisher-White, True Blue Tattoo, Queens, NY)

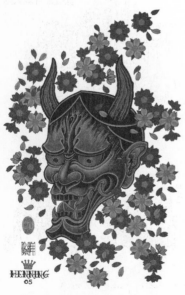

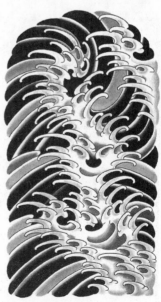

(Courtesy of Henning Jorgensen, Royal Tattoo, Helsignør, DK, www.royaltattoo.com)

(Courtesy of John Reardon, Saved Tattoo, Brooklyn, NY, www.johnreardontattoos.com)

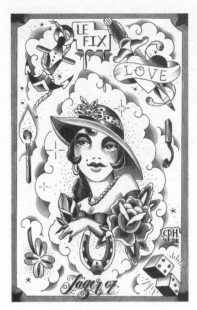

(Courtesy of Franz Jager, LeFix Tattoo, Copenhagen, DK, www.le-fix.com)

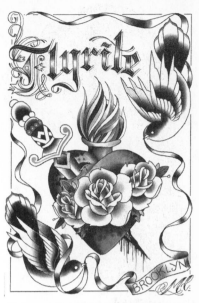

(Courtesy of Marina Inoue, Flyrite Tattoo, Brooklyn, NY, www.flyritetattoo.net)

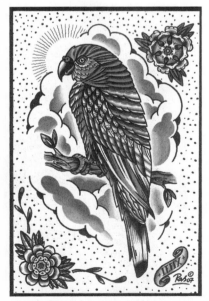

(Courtesy of Ras, LeFix Tattoo, Copenhagen, DK, www.le-fix.com)

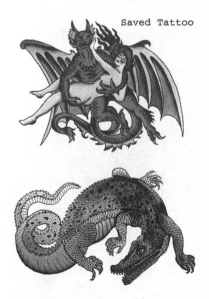

(Courtesy of Michelle Tarantelli, Saved Tattoo, Brooklyn, NY, www.savedtattoo.com)

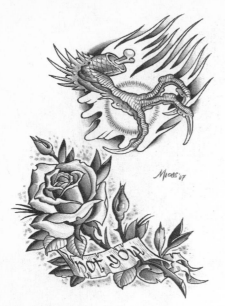

(Courtesy of Midas, Cobra Custom Tattoo, Plymouth, MA, cobracustomtattoo.com)

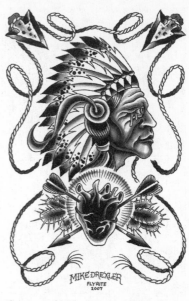

(Courtesy of Mike Drexler, Flyrite Tattoo, Brooklyn, NY, www.flyritetattoo.net)

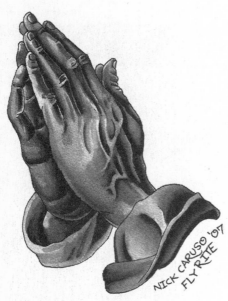

(Courtesy of Nick Caruso, Flyrite Tattoo, Brooklyn, NY, www.flyritetattoo.net)

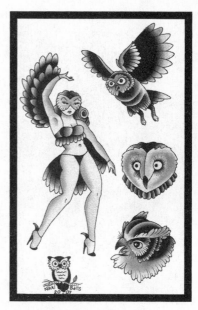

(Courtesy of Nikki Balls, Tattoo Paradise, Wheaton, MD, www.tattooparadisedc.com)

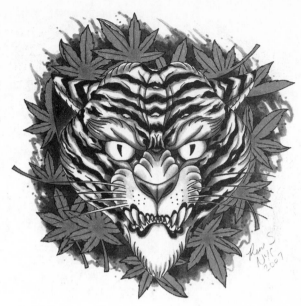

(Courtesy of Rene Santiago,
Inkman Tattoo, Brooklyn, NY,
www.myspace.com/renesantiagotatuajes

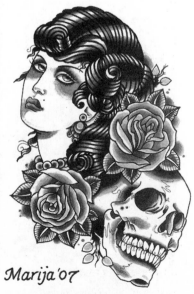

Marija'07

(Courtesy of Marija Asanovski,
Royal Tattoo, Helsignør, DK,
www.royaltattoo.com)

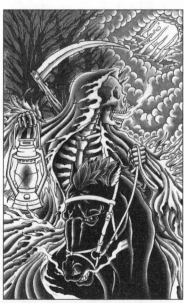

(Courtesy of Rene Santiago,
Inkman Tattoo, Brooklyn, NY,
www.myspace.com/renesantiagotatuajes

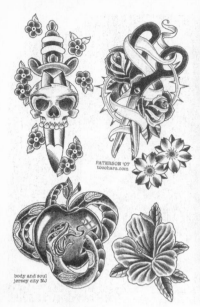

(Courtesy of Adam Paterson, Body and Soul Tattoo, Jersey City, NJ, www.tocohara.com)

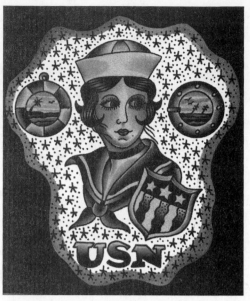

(Courtesy of Daniel Santoro, NYC, www.teenageghosts.com)

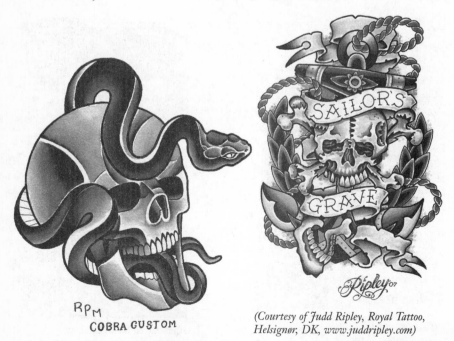

(Courtesy of Ryan MacNamara, Cobra Custom Tattoo, Plymouth, MA, cobracustomtattoo.com)

(Courtesy of Judd Ripley, Royal Tattoo, Helsignør, DK, www.juddripley.com)

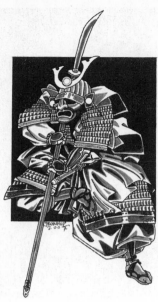

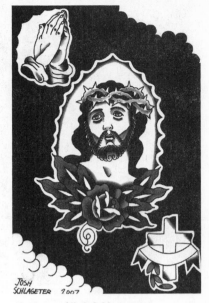

(Courtesy of Steve Huie,
Flyrite Tattoo, Brooklyn, NY,
www.flyritetattoo.net)

(Courtesy of Josh Schlageter,
H.O.D Tattoo, Buffalo, NY)

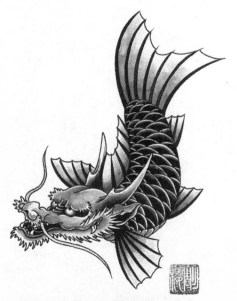

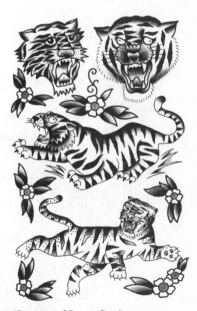

(Courtesy of Shinji [Horizakura],
New York Adorned, Brooklyn, NY,
www.nyadorned.com)

(Courtesy of Stacey Gardiner,
Frith Street Tattoo, London,
England. www.myspace.com/
xbugsxstaceyxtattoosx)

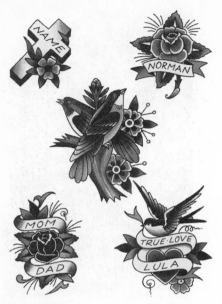

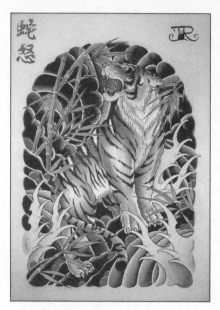

(Courtesy of Steve Boltz, Brooklyn, NY, www.steveboltz.com)

(Courtesy of Judd Ripley, Royal Tattoo, Helsingør, DK, www.juddripley.com)

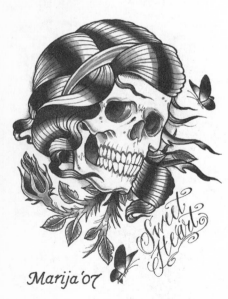

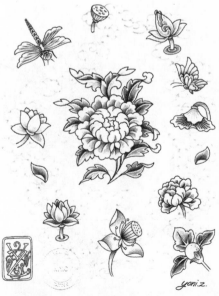

(Courtesy of Marija Asanovski, Royal Tattoo, Helsingør, DK, www.royaltattoo.com)

(Courtesy of Yoni Zilber, New York Adorned, www.yoniztattoo.com)

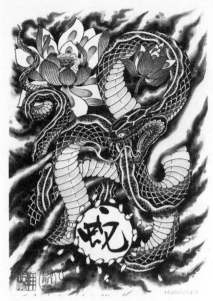

*(Courtesy of Henning Jorgensen,
Royal Tattoo, Helsignør, DK,
www.royaltattoo.com)*

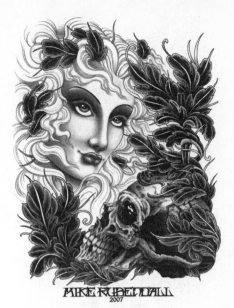

*(Courtesy of Mike Rubendall,
Kings Avenue Tattoo, N. Massapequa, NY,
kingsavenuetattoo.com. Photo courtesy of
Skullproject.com)*

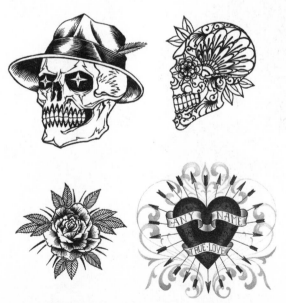

*(Courtesy of Scott Campbell, Saved Tattoo, Brooklyn, NY,
www.savedtattoo.com)*

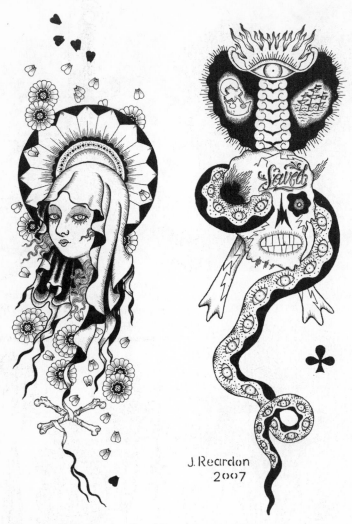

(Courtesy of John Reardon, Saved Tattoo, Brooklyn, NY,
www.johnreardontattoos.com)

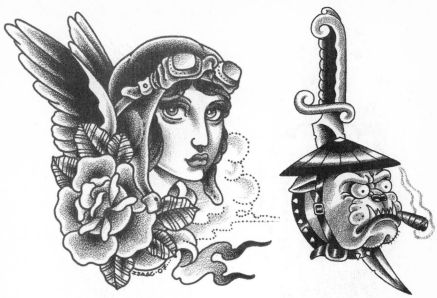

(Courtesy of Isaac Fainkujen, Tempe, AZ)

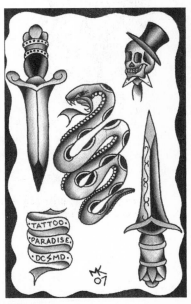

(Courtesy of Aaron Coleman, Immaculate Tattoo, Mesa, AZ)

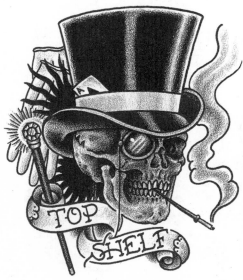

(Courtesy of Shag, Black Luck Studios, Phoenix, AZ)

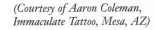

(Courtesy of Matt Knopp, Tattoo Paradise, Washington DC, www.tattooparadisedc.com)

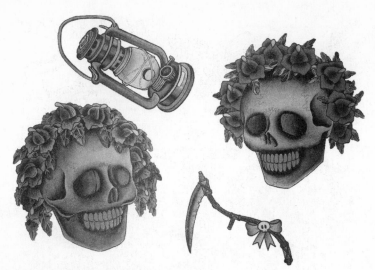

(Courtesy of Amina Reardon, Tato Svend, Copenhagen, DK, www.tato-svend.dk)

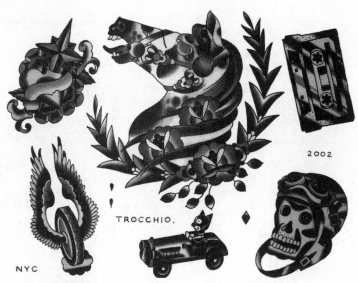

(Courtesy of Dan Trocchio, Saved Tattoo, Brooklyn, NY, www.myspace.com/danieltrocchio)

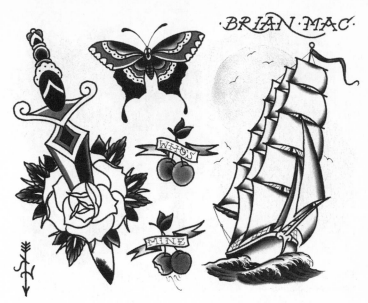

(Courtesy of Brian Mac, Cobra Custom Tattoo, Plymouth, MA, cobracustomtattoo.com)

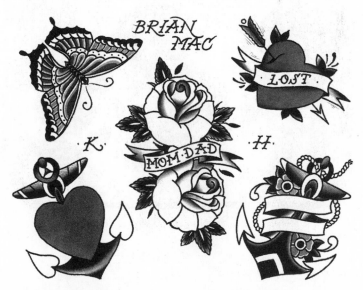

(Courtesy of Brian Mac, Cobra Custom Tattoo, Plymouth, MA, cobracustomtattoo.com)

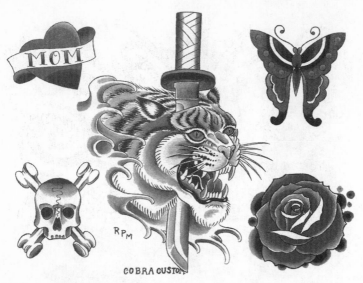

(Courtesy of Ryan MacNamara, Cobra Custom Tattoo, Plymouth, MA, cobracustomtattoo.com)

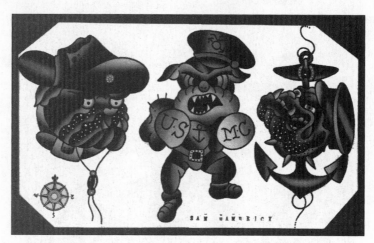

(Courtesy of Sam Hambrick, Immortal Ink Tattoos, Clinton, NJ, www.sweettatsbro.com)

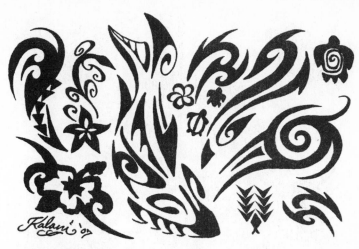

(Courtesy of Kalani Kelly, Liquid Metal Tattoo, Aiea, HI, www.kalanitattoo.com)

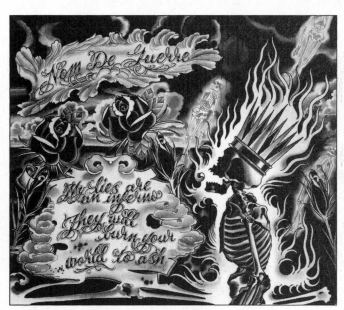

(Courtesy of Dan Trocchio, Saved Tattoo, Brooklyn, NY, www.myspace.com/danieltrocchio)

Where to Look for Tattooists and Designs

Online and Magazine Resources

Google: Search the word "tattoos" or "tattoo": www.google.com

MySpace: www.myspace.com/guidetogettingatattoo

Tattoos.com: www.tattoos.com

Tattoo Archive: www.tattooarchive.com

Tattoo Collector Magazine: www.tattoocollectormagazine.com

Revenant Publishing: www.revenantpublishing.com

Old Ghosts: www.oldghostsflash.com

Prick Magazine: www.prickmag.net

International Tattoo

Tattoo Magazine

Juxtapose

Tattoo Artist Magazine

Tattoo Life   Skin & Ink

Tattoo Energy   Tattoo

Flash Books and Recommended Reading

Old Ghosts, A flash Collection. Revenant Publishing, 2005.

Bella. Revenant Publishing, 2007.

Revisited. A Tribute to Flash From the Past. Revenant Publishing, 2007.

Skull Project. www.skullproject.com, Mathew Amy, 2007.

Sailor Jerry Tattoo Flash, Second Edition. Don Ed Hardy, Hardy Marks Publications, 2007.

Sailor Jerry Tattoo Flash (Volume 2). Don Ed Hardy, Hardy Marks Publications, 2004.

The New York City Tattoo: The Oral History of an Urban Art. Michael McCabe, Hardy Marks Publications, 1997.

Japanese Tattooing Now. Michael McCabe, Schiffer Publications, 2004.

Tattoos of Indochina. Michael McCabe, Schiffer Publications, 2002.

Tattooing New York City. Michael McCabe, Schiffer Publications, 1999.

Tattoo History. Steve Gilbert, Juno Books, 2000.

Legacy: The Horiyoshi III Tradition. Juan Puente, 2006.

Tattooing from Japan to the West. Takahiro Kitamura, Schiffer Publishing, 2005.

Bushido: Legacies of the Japanese Tattoo. Takahiro Kitamura and Katie M. Kitamura, Schiffer Publishing, 2001.

Russian Criminal Tattoo Encyclopedia. Danzig Baldaev and Sergei Vasiliev and Alexei Plutser-Sarno, Steidl/Fuel, 2003.

Haunted. Dave Fox, PrestoArt, 2005.

Tattooing the Invisible Man, Second Edition. Don Ed Hardy, Hardy Marks Publications, 2007.

True Love Tattoos. Henk Schiffmacher, Taschen, 2001.

Index